TREATING PEOPLE
WITH CHRONIC DISEASE

TREATING PEOPLE WITH CHRONIC DISEASE: A PSYCHOLOGICAL GUIDE

CAROL D. GOODHEART, EdD
AND
MARTHA H. LANSING, MD

AMERICAN PSYCHOLOGICAL ASSOCIATION
WASHINGTON, DC

First printing November 1996
Second printing June 1997

Published by
American Psychological Association
750 First Street, NE
Washington, DC 20002

Copies may be ordered from
APA Order Department
P.O. Box 92984
Washington, DC 20090-2984

In the United Kingdom and Europe, copies may be ordered from
American Psychological Association
3 Henrietta Street
Covent Garden, London
WC2E 8LU England

Printer: Data Reproductions Corp., Rochester Hills, MI
Typesetter: Innodata, Hanover, MD
Cover Designer: Minker Design, Bethesda, MD
Technical/Production Editor: Ida Audeh

Library of Congress Cataloging-in-Publication Data
Goodheart, Carol D.
       Treating people with chronic disease: a psychological guide /
    Carol D. Goodheart and Martha H. Lansing.
          p.   cm. —— (Psychologists in independent practice book series)
       Includes bibliographical references and index.
       ISBN 1-55798-387-9
       1. Chronic diseases—Psychological aspects.   2. Sick—Psychology.
    3. Chronically ill—Mental health.   I. Lansing, Martha H.
    II. Title.   III. Series.
       [DNLM: 1. Chronic Disease—therapy.   2. Chronic Disease—
    psychology.   3. Psychotherapy.   WT 500 G652t 1996]
       RC108.G66   1996
    616'.001'9—dc20
    DNLM/DLC
    for Library of Congress
                                                                                96-30817
                                                                                      CIP

British Library Cataloguing in Publication Data
A CIP record is available from the British Library.

Printed in the United States of America

To our families, in sickness and in health
Hugh
Leigh, Pamela, Rebecca
Richard, Michael, Robert
Katherine, Emily
Bridget, Michael
Pat and Rubby

Carol Goodheart

✣ ✣ ✣

Douglas
Elizabeth, Carolyn, Stephen
Ed
Ruth
in memory of Betty

Martha Lansing

Contents

Preface

This book is a collaboration by two members of different professions, psychology and medicine; each of us has a distinct voice and view, but we have a shared vision. By training and inclination, we are both practitioners and psychoanalysts, and we bring that background to the treatment of patients with chronic physical illness. Each of us traveled along a different route, yet reached a common vantage point. We have found the dynamic collaborative view to be stronger, sounder, and richer than we could have achieved alone, and we hope that both psychologists and physicians benefit from the sharing and interweaving of perspectives.

Carol D. Goodheart is a practicing, teaching, and supervising psychologist who started the project with a simple plan for writing about the treatment of patients with ambiguous waxing and waning diseases. Initially, that seemed to be distinct from her work with breast cancer patients, a population that, in turn, seemed different from her patients with steady-state diabetes. The project was put on hold for a year when a child in her family was diagnosed with cancer. The world of radical pediatric oncology treatment and its impact on several generations of family became more personal than professional. At the same time, the experience provided a dimension not obtainable by any other means. Sick patients and their relatives talked to the author as a fellow traveler about their needs, feelings, and experiences, without the formality and hesitation often accorded the professional. The result was the stirrings of a more comprehensive view of chronic illness that would encompass the waxing and waning diseases, the cancers, and the more steady-state diseases.

Martha H. Lansing is a board-certified family physician. Early in her practice of medicine, she realized the importance of communicating with psychologists about mutual patients. She became deeply interested in the way the mind interacts with the body in sickness and in health. She chose further training in psychoanalysis rather than in psychiatry to expand her view beyond the medical model. Today she maintains both a medical and a psychotherapy practice. In the course of her training, she came to know Carol Goodheart as both a teacher and a supervising analyst.

As we worked together, we began to share the treatment of patients with chronic illness in the community, and we developed a working psychologist–physician model. Out of this learning–teaching–discussing matrix came the collaboration that became the book.

The book is written from our clinical experience and contains many stories, examples, and vignettes about patients we have known and treated and whose treatment we have supervised. All of the patients presented throughout the book have been disguised to protect their identities, but the illustrations of the point under discussion remain clinically accurate. Outcomes for any specific patients given do not necessarily reflect the course or outcome that may be expected for other patients.

We have chosen the term *patient* to represent people with chronic illnesses, because it is a term common to the disciplines of both medicine and psychology. Several people with illnesses have told us they do not like being referred to as patients, because it categorizes them in a limited role. Mindful of this, we have attempted to use general social terms when appropriate and to use the term *patient* as an identifier, just as we have used the identifying term *therapist*. It is not our intent to label people, but rather to present clinical material in a clear and consistent style.

Some readers who are also therapists will have chronic diseases themselves, in which case the book may be read as a resource for helping others and oneself. We expect that these therapists will be an instrumental force in adding to our work by contributing new ideas and approaches for the psychological treatment of people with chronic illness.

We would like to express our appreciation to our patients for the opportunity to participate in their lives and to learn from them.

Acknowledgments

Many family members, friends, colleagues, and patients have influenced our thinking about chronic illness. In particular, we appreciate the contributions of the following individuals: Leigh A. Woznick, for being the researcher and resource guide par excellence; Sandra Haber, PhD, for being such a sensitive reader, commentator, and global thinker; Myron Gessner, MD, Anne Kayzak, PhD, and Richard Womer, MD, for their knowledge, research, and care of ill children; Hugh R. Goodheart, for computer expertise, technical manuscript preparation, and encouragement during the hardest moments; Douglas Lansing, for inspiration and unfailing support; The PsychHealth, P.A. partners: Melanie Callender, PhD, Ora Gourarie, PsyD, Owen Isaacs, EdD, Phyllis Marganoff, EdD, and Jeffrey Pusar, PsyD, for the group support to develop the Health Project; Donald Spence, PhD, for the expression of an analytic voice; Barbara Galione, for manuscript assistance; and the Division of Independent Practice, American Psychological Association, for giving our project a home.

I

Understanding Chronic Illness

1

Introduction to Chronic Illness: A Holographic View

With increasing frequency, psychotherapy practitioners encounter patients who struggle with enduring physical illnesses. These chronic illnesses make up a spectrum of diseases. Some are life threatening, such as cancer, cardiovascular disease, and AIDS; some are understood and manageable, such as diabetes and hypertension; some are understood but progressively disabling, such as hearing and vision loss associated with aging; and some are poorly understood and unpredictable, such as arthritis, multiple sclerosis, and chronic fatigue syndrome. All of these chronic illnesses have a common psychological thread: The individual will never again return to the pre-illness sense of self, of options, of invulnerability, of obliviousness to the body's functioning.

The patients are sick. They are not getting better, and they may get worse, which creates a psychological conundrum for people living in a sophisticated technological era. There is a fundamental dichotomy between the expectations of a technological society, which promise solutions and cures for problems, and the reality of chronic debilitating illness, which fosters confusion and regression to the superstitious magical thinking of the past.[1]

---

[1]*Magical thinking*, a term used repeatedly throughout the book, involves several overlapping elements that contribute to its special properties. These include enchantment, superstition, fantasy, the supernatural, and the distortion of elements of reality for the purposes of wish fulfillment.

Patients come to psychotherapy with self-doubts and fears that they will not be understood; they struggle to regain control over their bodies, lives, and perceptions of reality. All of these forces interact with patients' premorbid personality structures and their level of defensive and adaptive resources.

The individual's strongest wish is to return to "normal." Often, the psychotherapist's strongest wish is to heal. Nevertheless, the range of possibilities on the psychobiological spectrum is bewildering. Continuing physical disability forces the alteration of the patient's basic life functions and routines. The symptoms may interfere with the ability to work, to carry out family roles, to play, and to rest, all to varying degrees. As a disease persists, symptoms may be constant at times (which is discouraging and frightening), lessened or in remission at times (which stirs hope), unpredictably erratic at times (which is maddening and frustrating), or relentlessly progressive (which is exhausting and overwhelming). As disability and ambiguity persist, a significant internal psychological disorganization begins. A challenge to the established sense of self arises. The uncertainty, progression, and unpredictability of illness create anxiety in the therapist as well as in the patient.

Falvo (1991, p. 2) outlined a series of the potential threats of illness that are useful to consider:

- ☐ threats to life and physical well-being;
- ☐ threats to body integrity and comfort (result of disease, treatment, or procedures);
- ☐ threats to independence, privacy, autonomy, and control;
- ☐ threats to self-concept and fulfillment of customary roles;
- ☐ threats to life goals and future plans;
- ☐ threats to relationships with family, friends, colleagues;
- ☐ threats to ability to remain in familiar surroundings; and
- ☐ threats to economic well-being.

The degree of threat may vary from patient to patient, but the actual identified factors are quite comprehensive, and clinicians may expect to encounter them frequently when treating patients with chronic illness.

The adaptive goal of psychotherapy for these patients (the desired outcome) is the stability of self and identity in the face of the body's instability and uncertain course. One may use many strategies to reach that goal, but any successful strategy must address two related factors: (a) the overarching problem of internal disorganization that threatens the structure of the self and identity; and (b) the building process of reorganization, a reconsolidation of self and identity, based on a changed reality.

Serving the Underserved

People with chronic physical illnesses are an underserved population who require the services of both psychologists and physicians in their own communities. Many of the great medical centers throughout the nation offer sophisticated programs for their patients. However, patients who receive psychological services in institutional settings from health specialists are frequently left to flounder when they return home. Most patients receive medical treatment and follow-up in their local community, but they receive no psychological treatment at all. We believe psychological treatment should be integrated as a part of routine disease management. It should not be left as an afterthought or a stopgap response to a crisis, offered to patients only when they break down, lose control, or make life difficult for those around them.

Cardiac rehabilitation opportunities for patients offer a telling example of community need. In a press conference, the Agency for Health Care Policy and Research released findings from a 2-year study of supervised cardiac rehabilitation programs. One startling result showed that fewer than one third of heart patients participated in the programs. Such programs typically offer individualized diet and exercise regimens, stress reduction, smoking cessation, and other health-promoting practices. Part of the difficulty with utilization for these programs lies in their location. The independent panel called for more accessible sites in the community, not just the medical centers (Leary, October 11, 1995).

The government agency assembled a 19-member panel to produce the study (Wenger et al., 1995). It included consumers and professionals from the fields of medicine, nursing, psychology, exercise physiology, nutrition, and physical and occupational therapy. Unfortunately, the publication guideline described counseling and behavioral interventions in limited terms. *Counseling* was defined as "providing advice, support, and consultation"; *behavioral interventions* were defined as "systematic instruction in techniques to modify health-related behaviors" (p. 16). A broader psychological context for definitions might have contributed key dimensions that affect the utilization of these programs, namely, individual and systems psychology (e.g., personality, resistance, habit strengths, compulsions, defenses, personal and family dynamics, beliefs, mores, and the impact of economic pressures). Given the prevalence of heart disease, it is important that health care professionals help patients understand, work through, and take advantage of strategies and resources for better management of their disease.

General psychotherapy practitioners do not ordinarily view themselves as health practitioners, but rather as mental health practitioners. Most community-based psychologists are not sufficiently educated in health psychology to feel comfortable with offering specialty treatment. Nevertheless, the need for broad-based community psychological services remains. Psychotherapists in independent practice seem to ignore chronic illness for several reasons: (a) lack of training and the erroneous assumption that patients' needs are being met by health care specialists; (b) frank distaste and anxiety in the face of protracted illness; and (c) lack of medical knowledge or working relationships with physicians, nurses, physical therapists, and other health care providers. We hope this volume serves as a training tool, decreases aversion to working with the population, and encourages more collaboration and integration among the medical and psychological professional communities. Our primary goal is to prepare community-based practitioners to offer more effective psychological treatment to people with chronic physical illness.

Over the past few years, we have found an increase in these types of patients in our own psychotherapy practices and have witnessed an explosion of articles in the mass media and the scientific literature on the array of diseases and immune system dysfunctions and their correlation with stress. In the chapters that follow, we have attempted to translate overlapping medical and psychological information and to build a bridge that connects medicine and psychology, body and mind, in practical ways.

A Holographic View of Illness

Holography is derived from the Greek word "holos," meaning whole. It is a method used to create a three-dimensional image, which is an improvement over a flat two-dimensional image and enhances the visual field available for experience. The creation of a hologram of illness is our metaphor and model for the different views, angles, and dimensions that form the substance of the distinct chapters. When brought together in a projection that shows the interactive interference pattern of light beams, the resulting holographic image is far richer and fuller than any of the single or flat views alone. When brought together, the different views of illness also should form a more complete picture than any of the component parts alone.

Several points of information about holograms have been relevant to our model of illness. First, holography records the whole message of a light wave (Hecht, 1988). In other words, the hologram contains a whole picture of an object. Only the intensity of a light wave, not its cycle phase, is recorded by the human eye or photographic film. The creation of a hologram requires the mixing of two beams from one light source: an object beam (which is altered by the contact with an object) and a reference beam (which is unaltered). Hecht explained that it seems a simpler process than it actually is, because of technical problems involved in keeping the waves in both beams in proper phase with each other. The same may be said of illness and response to illness; keeping all views in mind can be a daunting project.

Second, holograms can store large amounts of data, and data storage can be multiplied even further by adding many holograms on top of each other (Bains, 1990). The system is not merely additive, but also performs logic operations on data, allowing a more accurate picture in which corresponding bits reinforce each other and out-of-phase bits cancel each other out.

Thus, the whole entity, the hologram of illness in our model, is shaped and refined by new and changing information.

Third, one may compare holograms of an object that are taken under different conditions, for example, before and after stress has been applied (Hecht, 1988). When viewed together, these holograms reveal where an object deforms under pressure. This process, which is called *holographic interferometry*, has been used in the testing of airplane tires to detect flaws. Tires are good if they change shape uniformly under pressure; they are apt to fail if they have weak points that are demonstrated by uneven changes in shape. The comparison of holograms of illness may also yield valuable information on the vulnerabilities of an individual, the weak points, and the pressure spots caused or affected by disease.

Overview of the Book

Each chapter gives a different view of illness and takes a different vantage point. Each chapter alone provides an important but incomplete view for the psychophysiological whole picture. Because each patient and therapist is different, it will be a matter of trial and experiment for the reader to examine the various views and to assemble them into an accurate hologram for a particular treatment situation.

In the first section of the book, we present a holographic model of illness consisting of four templates:

1. A **Medical Template** frames the disease.
2. A **Threat Template** shows a continuum of disease severity.
3. A **Response Template** shows a continuum of awareness and adaptation to disease.
4. A **Psychological Template** frames personality structure and functioning.

Chapter 2 introduces the nonphysician psychotherapy practitioner to a model for understanding disease: how to think about disease, what questions to ask, and how to locate a patient within the model. It is designed to shed light on the demand characteristics of a disease process. Categories of questions are organized under two templates, each of which carries different psychological implications. The Medical Template helps explain the disease itself; the Threat Template helps one assess the danger to existence posed by the disease. Together, these templates provide a perspective that gives the first holographic view of the patient with the chronic illness. The language for discussing disease is readily usable for dialogue with medical professionals, because it is based on a common medical framework for physician–patient discussion.

Chapter 3 focuses on the patient's response to illness and search for help. The Response Template continuum shows a typical progression of events, as well as modifying factors that must be taken into account. The internal process of assault to the established sense of self and the struggle to avoid the disorganizing experience are highlighted. A second holographic view is created by focusing on the experience-near[2] dimension of the patient's response to the unique press of a disease process.

Chapter 4 discusses the patient's premorbid personality organization, which includes both level of functioning and style of relating to people and navigating life's challenges. The Psychological Template of questions is presented as a guide for the assessment of a patient's characteristic ways of responding to stressors. The understanding of personality structure is an essential part of forming a basis for an effective treatment plan. In holography terms, the personality structure is close to the response to illness, but it is not identically positioned. There is a discernibly different angle of view, resulting in another holographic image. Thus, another dimension is added.

In the second section of the book, we turn to the applications of the templates to chronic illness, beginning with chapter 5 on psychological treatment. The purpose in developing a multidimensioned hologram of illness, with views of disease, response, structure, and disorganization process projected together, is to provide depth of information. A full in-depth picture is necessary for the selection, development, and assembling of truly

---

[2]*Experience-near* means *close to experience*. The concept of experience-near phenomenology is related to introspection, empathy, and the subjective internal representational world. It is derived from the work of Klein (1976), with subsequent elaborations by Stolorow and Atwood (1979).

therapeutic treatment approaches. An overview of the shared tasks of the patient and psychotherapist, treatment strategies, the match between focus of intervention and need, and a menu of interventions are discussed. Clinical examples of treatment focus are presented.

Countertransference is the subject of chapter 6. Countertransference issues, stirrings, and problems are part of the landscape of any psychotherapy. There are, however, some particularly noteworthy induced responses to the uncertainty, ambiguity, and losses that accompany illness. Special problems include the psychotherapist's own body anxieties and the universal phenomenon of death anxiety.

Chapter 7 opens up the interaction between the illness and the patient's world. Factors such as history, diversity, environment, role, and life stage have an impact on the psychological treatment. Nontraditional therapeutic approaches for a man with asthma and an adolescent with leukemia provide supporting clinical examples.

Children and adolescents with chronic illness are the focus of chapter 8. Because children are developing physically, emotionally, and cognitively and have not yet reached a maturely formed self and identity, the treatment model and task emphasis that are appropriate for adult patients must be altered. Our approach emphasizes multiple approaches for multiple problems, with a goal of fostering security and natural development to the greatest extent possible. To illustrate, we provide clinical examples of children with cancer and trauma resolution and children with diabetes and a coping paradigm. We include the stage of adolescence with a developmental emphasis and present the case of a teenager with cystic fibrosis. Treatment is based on the principle that the best approach depends much more on the child than the disease.

Chapter 9 expands the realm of illness to the context of the family system, both near and extended. This consideration of family examines interpersonal support systems overall and as specifically related to the chronically ill patient. Families both provide and require support themselves, especially when the impact of illness becomes a serious burden on caretaking family members. Chapter 10 tells the story of a young woman's illness, kidney transplant, and subsequent psychotherapy. The strides and limitations encountered in her psychotherapy provide an overview and a summary of the templates and concepts established in the foregoing chapters.

The third section of the book focuses on resources. The compendium of information provided in chapter 11 may be the most helpful section of all for a busy practitioner. Information on specific diseases and support services for patients and families is readily available through national disease organizations and government agencies. Many of these groups are listed, along with a brief description of the services provided. We have inquired about specific information on psychosocial issues for each resource, and such resources are noted, where available. The information may be accessed by the Internet, fax, telephone, or mail.

We hope we have provided a multidimensional view of the patient with chronic illness and have pointed the reader in directions that will be helpful when providing psychotherapy for this underserved group of people. Such terms as *rainbow holograms*, *alcove holograms*, and *multiplex holograms* point to the richness still to be expanded and explored in the world of holography. As holography still holds promise for greater development, so does psychotherapy for improved understanding and treatment of patients with chronic disease.

2

The Medical Template and the Threat Template: The Disease Perspective

Disease disturbs. It interferes with the normal vital physiological and psychological processes of the afflicted individual. Foremost in a sick person's mind may be the question of mortality: "Will I die?" More often, the most important question is one of duration: "How long will I be sick, out of work, in pain, disabled?" If the answer is a few days, weeks, or even a few months, most people can tolerate the disturbance in some way as they anticipate healing and a return to health. Illness that is limited and results in a return to normal functioning is classified as an *acute illness*.

Some illnesses, however, persist over months and years and never go away. Diseases may begin acutely and strongly, or they may begin with subliminal soft signs. There may be periods of remission, during which the person feels free of disease but is aware that the malady or its potential for recurrence or exacerbation remain. There may be no respite as the sickness pursues a relentless course, ending in profound disability or death. These long-standing diseases that forever alter normal physiological functioning are classified as *chronic illnesses*.

A single psychotherapist in a general practice may find a wide variety of chronic physical problems among his or her patients, such as heart disease and hypertension, infertility, breast cancer and prostate cancer, chronic fatigue syndrome, scleroderma, multiple sclerosis, diabetes, and all the problems of aging from deafness and lameness to Alzheimer's disease. Chronic illnesses and conditions are myriad, and thinking about these illnesses can become very confusing indeed for psychotherapists, patients, and even for physicians.

We have found it useful to think about chronic illness in several ways, which we have organized into templates. Each template is a gauge, a guide to categorize and understand any particular illness and its expected or potential disturbance of the affected person's vitality.

The Medical Template	The Threat Template
□ Outcome	□ Life Threatening
□ Process	□ Progressive
□ Etiology	□ Unpredictable
□ Needs	□ Manageable

The Medical Template opens the door to understanding the disease itself. It categorizes disease by outcome, process, etiology, and management needs (OPEN). The questions posed in this medical template can be used by psychologists and patients alike to obtain a clear understanding of the nature of an illness from physicians and other health care professionals. In fact, physicians often use a similar format when they explain illness to patients, family members, employers, and psychotherapists. The references listed at the end of this book include a set of medical references that can be found in most hospital and medical center libraries and are accessible to practitioners working with patients with chronic illness. One of these volumes, *The Merck Manual of Diagnosis and Therapy* (Berkow & Fletcher, 1992), is inexpensive and should be part of an individual practitioner's personal library.

The Threat Template does not lend itself to a handy acronym, but it provides essential information that is not available with the use of the medical template alone. The questions of this template give one a sense of the threat a disease poses to an individual, both for existence itself and for his or her accustomed way of living. The Threat Template categorizes chronic diseases as life threatening; as understood, but progressively disabling; as poorly understood and unpredictable; and finally, as understood and manageable. The categories derive from information obtained by using the Medical Template. For example, one has to consider the outcomes for particular diseases before one can judge the threat to life. Cancer is a frightening disease that many people assume is always life threatening. Nevertheless, there are variable expectations for outcome, even within subcategories: Certain types of skin cancer are almost always curable; other skin cancers are present but indolent for years without disabling progression; still others, such as malignant melanoma, can follow a virulent course and lead to death within a few months of initial diagnosis. Physicians may not be able to give exact predictions, but they are often able to tell psychotherapy practitioners what outcome is expected. In the same vein, physicians can offer an assessment of manageability based on expectations about the medical management and treatment choices for the specific disease. Again, the medical references at the end of this book can help one determine where a particular patient with a particular disease falls on the threat to life and lifestyle continuum.

The two sets of categories for the Medical Template and the Threat Template yield information that leads to different psychological implications. A particular disease may have different presentations. The templates can be used to evaluate the disease for the individual patient concerned. The response to the template questions will not be the same for every patient with a given disease. For example, diabetes is generally manageable, even when patients are dependent on insulin. For some individuals, however, diabetes can be totally out of control. These individuals may have kidney failure and heart failure and face death within months. Thus, patients may have the same chronic disease, diabetes, but different psychological problems to pursue. Some patients must adapt to an altered lifestyle of following blood sugars and taking medication for the rest of their lives; others must think about dying in the near future and planning for that event. A psychotherapist who is working with diabetic patients must understand these most basic differences (Griffith & Dambro, 1994, p. 289).

Furthermore, a disease can change its presentation over time. One of our patients had ovarian cancer and had been in remission for 15 years. After all that time, she developed a metastasis and became profoundly ill and debilitated. For this patient, the disease process, outcome, and management needs had changed radically. The disease had changed from being understood and manageable to being life threatening; she ultimately succumbed to a disease that she believed had been cured. Periodically, patients and psychotherapists should use the templates to reassess the status of a disease. Reassessment can provide new directions for understanding and treating patients with chronic illness.

The Medical Template: "OPEN"

This system of thinking about disease poses four questions:

- □ What is the outcome of the disease?
- □ What is the disease process?
- □ What is the etiology of the disease?
- □ What are the expected management needs?

The OPEN template provides information about the physiological environment and the demand characteristics of a disease. It is important to note that disease is an always changing, never static phenomenon.

Outcome

Outcome may be expressed in terms of known versus unknown, cure versus death, or level and type of disability. Perhaps the most honest assessment of disease outcome is that it is unknown. Even in instances of high statistical probabilities for outcome, one cannot predict with certainty. For example, if a woman with a particular form of ovarian cancer has only a 5% chance of survival, how does one know whether she will become one of the fortunate survivors or whether she will be one of the 95% for whom the disease is terminal? Of course, for most cancers the statistical probabilities are not so extreme.

For many diseases, the expectations for outcome are much more ambiguous. Despite the advances of modern medicine, there are many diseases so poorly understood that little is known about their progression and outcome. Over time, physicians may come to understand these diseases and to better predict the outcome, but at present they are still puzzles. One such puzzle is presented by Lyme disease.

In the 1970s, the medical community was aware of an illness associated with enlarged lymph nodes, a strange "bull's eye" rash, swollen joints that "migrated" (e.g., one day a wrist would be swollen, the next day a knee would be the affected site). In fact, the rash had been known for many years as "chronicum migrans." Gradually, Lyme disease has come to be understood as the result of the *Borrelia burgdorferi* spirochete bacteria that is deposited into the human body through a tick bite. Once infected, the body sets up multiple reactions to rid itself of the invading organisms; these reactions produce the symptoms of rash, swollen glands, fever, migratory joint pain, and malaise (Sigal et al., 1993).

In the 1980s, the disease gained notoriety as it spread throughout the country, infecting more and more people. Many physicians began to treat their patients with stronger and larger doses of antibiotics to help the body fight the organism. Some patients were diagnosed quickly and accurately and were treated successfully. Other patients never developed the tell-tale identifying rash and were carrying the symptoms of joint pain and debilitating fatigue for months until they were correctly diagnosed and began treatment. Still others were diagnosed when the spirochete moved from the bloodstream into the central nervous system, producing symptoms such as facial palsy. Some patients recovered completely with treatment, whereas others languished despite months of intravenous antibiotic therapy.

By the 1990s, the term *post-Lyme syndrome* had been coined. The syndrome, which is still poorly understood, leaves patients in a weakened state, often with arthritis and other physical complaints. No one knows why these patients have not recovered fully or whether they ever will. Physicians are frequently pressed by patients and their families to try more antibiotics, even after the recommended course is completed. Conversely, many health care providers (physicians and psychologists alike) do not take the patients' symptoms seriously. They dismiss patients as simply depressed or psychosomatic. Contributing to the puzzle is the commonly noticed depressive element. Depression can be associated with both the aftermath of an infectious process and the chronic struggles of daily living when a person feels ill. In fact, some patients are helped by antidepressant medications. Others do not respond. Eventually, these nonresponders may be labeled *psychosomatic*. The secrets of Lyme disease and post-Lyme syndrome may be uncovered in the future. It is difficult to accept the fact that for many patients, the outcome remains unknown (Wyngaarden, Smith, & Bennett, 1992, pp. 1772–1777).

Many other diseases, including rheumatoid arthritis, systemic lupus, chronic fatigue syndrome, and multiple sclerosis, present unknown outcomes. Another subset of diseases has modifying clauses attached to the question of outcome, because treatment or lifestyle change may alter the outcome. Hypertension and diabetes are examples of modifiable diseases. If no medication or lifestyle changes are implemented, hypertension can lead to heart disease and stroke, which could be severely debilitating or fatal (Griffith & Dambro, 1994, pp. 492, 493). This kind of modifiable disease does not carry an expectation of fatality, if it is properly treated and managed. Yet it remains largely unknown why some people, even with the requisite treatment and lifestyle changes, develop malignant hypertension and stroke, whereas others who remain untreated live a full life and ultimately die of an unrelated disease.

The most dramatic dimension for outcome is the threat to life. At one end of a continuum are illnesses that are essentially non-life threatening (e.g., irritable bowel syndrome). At the other end of the continuum are diseases that have no known cure and often end in death (e.g., AIDS). Many diseases (e.g., cardiovascular disease, diabetes) fall in between the poles of the continuum.

Surprisingly, the outcome of a chronic disease may not be continued chronicity, but rather, a cure. One does not expect cure in chronic diseases, but there are many stories of cure that turn expectations upside down. Rocky Mountain spotted fever is the focus for one such story. Before 1960, this fever was described in medical books and journals as having a progressive painful course, often culminating in death. However, in a literature search for materials published since 1960, no such description could be found. Why? The outcome for the disease changed dramatically during the 1950s with the discovery of the antibiotics tetracycline and chloramphenicol. Now curable, it is an acute illness that lasts approximately 2 weeks (Thoene, 1995, pp. 576–577).

Outcome is related also to types and levels of disability. For example, hearing loss may be minor or major, with abrupt or gradual changes, with onset in childhood, adulthood, or old age. In the progression of disability, there are often "tip" points in functioning, at which point the person is no longer able to maintain his or her previous life activities. When the magnitude of hearing loss became great enough for one 40-year-old man whom we treated, he could no longer use a telephone or go to the movies or out to a restaurant with friends, because he was unable to follow conversations. After three automobile accidents he stopped driving, for fear that his hearing loss was a contributing factor to the accidents. Because he was struggling at a "tip point," he became increasingly isolated and depressed. Psychotherapy was helpful to him in making the transition from a hearing to a nonhearing life, which involved coming to grips with his losses and learning new modes of access to the world (e.g., a telephone device for the deaf). Disability progression is a consideration for outcome; it is discussed in the next section.

Process

The process of disease may be described as (a) indolent (slow to grow or inactive), but progressive; (b) rapid, even violent; or (c) waxing and waning, with exacerbations and remissions. Although these categories overlap, they remain useful guidelines. Most of the processes we discuss may be altered (either speeded up or slowed down) by medical treatment and lifestyle changes or influenced by biological, psychological, and social factors.

Non–insulin-dependent diabetes is an example of an indolent but progressive disease. Early in the course of the diabetes, individuals are reminded of disease only by the need to monitor diet, exercise, and blood sugars. They do not ordinarily feel the disease. Those with diabetes often are not aware that small changes are occurring to nerves and blood vessels from day to day, month to month, and year to year. Because the process is not overt, it is very hard for many people who feel no changes in their bodies to persist in controlling diet, exercise, and blood sugars. As the disease progresses, diabetic individuals may need to introduce the use of medication and eventually the use of insulin. Even with the addition of medication, they are unlikely to feel the disease in the body. After many years, they will become aware of changes in vision or perhaps numbness in toes or fingers. These are signs that the disease is present and progressive and has been in the body for a long time (Wyngaarden et al., 1992, pp. 1291–1310).

The process of hypertension works similarly. Those with hypertension may feel little or nothing in their bodies. Their only awareness of the hypertension may come from an occasional elevated blood pressure reading. Once informed of the need for medication and monitoring, some people choose to ignore their disease process. They may refuse checkups, because they do not want to be reminded that disease is working in their bodies (Wyngaarden et al., 1992, pp. 253–269). For example, one attractive 40-year-old woman could not accept her diagnosis of hypertension, because it implied an imperfection in her body. Because she could "feel" nothing wrong, she ignored advice from her physician and family to take her medication and monitor her blood pressure. At the age of 51 she had a debilitating stroke, the result of arterial damage and high blood pressure, which left her unable to respond to her environment in any observable way.

Aging is accompanied by many symptoms, losses, and diseases that are indolent but progressive (e.g., loss of vision, loss of hearing, Parkinson's disease, and Alzheimer's disease). Often, there is no known way to stop the progression of indolent processes, but they may be speeded up or slowed down by medication or lifestyle changes. For example, the use of tobacco speeds the debilitating process of emphysema. Stopping tobacco smoking can slow the disease's rate of progression.

Some diseases proceed rapidly or violently (or both) from time of onset to final outcome. Particular kinds of ovarian cancers and some melanomas are relentless in their course, weakening the individual quickly. AIDS is a cruel disease; the patient suffers one episode of infection after another until the body is no longer able to respond and death ensues. Amyotrophic lateral sclerosis (Lou Gehrig's disease) can be so ruthless in its debilitating course that the sufferer is always aware of the disease process taking its body toll. Some forms of systemic lupus erythematosus and multiple sclerosis can be almost as violent because they incapacitate a person. Lupus can roar through a person, starting with painful arthritis; moving to kidney failure, heart and lung damage, and loss of brain function; and finally (mercifully) death—all within a year.

More often, systemic lupus erythematosus is among the disease processes that fall under the rubric of waxing and waning illnesses (Griffith & Dambro, 1994, pp. 974–975). Like the diseases of unknown outcome, these exacerbating and remitting diseases are perplexing to patients and their families, friends, and employers. One of our patients with lupus has periods of years in which she feels nothing unusual in her body. No laboratory or physical findings indicate problems. During these disease-free periods she does not require medication. Without warning, the disease flares suddenly with incapacitating arthritis. After several months of sophisticated medication regimens, the arthritis subsides, almost as abruptly as it appeared. For this woman, there is no way to predict either the outcome or the disease process. The safest prediction is that the disease will flare again.

The previously mentioned post-Lyme syndrome has a waxing and waning course, as do postpolio syndrome, multiple sclerosis, rheumatoid arthritis, and chronic fatigue syndrome. People spend much time, money, and energy trying to predict, prepare for, and prevent the exacerbations of their illnesses. Many cancers, such as the lymphomas and leukemias, can enter periods of remission following chemotherapy or irradiation treatment. People with these diseases have to live with the insecurity of not knowing whether they will remain free of cancer or whether the disease will recur.

Whatever the disease process—quiescent, creeping slowly, racing ahead, or ebbing and flowing—a psychological struggle to understand and control the illness is spawned. For each kind of disease, as for each individual, an understanding of the disease process can help the psychotherapist who works with the ill patient.

Etiology

The etiology category has meaningful psychological implications, which may be as important to the work of psychotherapy as is an understanding of disease outcome and process. The tracking of etiology takes into account whether the disease is of known origin, genetically determined, influenced by environment, influenced by behavior, or part of the natural aging process. Knowing or not knowing the cause and sources of disease creates different problems and anxieties for patients and their families.

A great deal is known about cardiovascular diseases. The anatomy and physiology of the system that includes the heart, the coronary arteries, and the extended arteries and veins are well understood, as are the diseases that result from problems within the system. Because the etiologies of cardiac and cardiovascular diseases are known, treatments for these diseases are well established. Sophisticated diagnostic techniques and treatment technologies are developed with regularity. Old tried and true strategies for reducing risk factors are well publicized. Of course, whether or not a person follows treatment and risk reduction recommendations is another matter, one that presents a concern for health psychologists, physicians, researchers, and public policy makers.

Contrast the known etiology of arteriosclerotic heart disease (Griffith & Dambro, 1994, pp. 72–73) with the unknown mysterious maze of information and misinformation surrounding chronic fatigue syndrome. During the 1980s several causes for this syndrome were postulated. As each new cause was announced, patients became excited at the prospect that discovery of the cause would lead to discovery of a cure. To date, however, none of the suggested causes of chronic fatigue syndrome have proven to be reliably verifiable. The physiological criteria for the syndrome are described and clear, but people debate the reality of the syndrome, because the etiology is unknown (Griffith & Dambro, 1994, p. 210).

There is a clear genetic predisposition for some diseases, and some gene markers have been identified. A family history of breast cancer or cardiovascular disease (e.g., coronary artery disease, hypertension, stroke, heart failure) is not an absolute predictor, but it is considered a sign of increased risk for the disease. The heritability factors for other cancers, Alzheimer's disease, and many other diseases are under investigation.

Some diseases have a marked genetic etiology; in Huntington's disease (chorea), for example, the abnormal gene is laid down at conception. The disease itself may not become evident until well into middle age. Genetic counseling is available at medical centers and other specialty sites to help families understand the nature of hereditary diseases. Such programs provide early diagnosis, identification of "carriers," and information on statistical prediction, which may be used for pregnancy and family planning (Thoene, 1995, pp. 310–311). Other genetically related disorders include hemophilia, certain types of muscular dystrophy, neurofibromatosis, sickle cell disease, and Down's syndrome.

Knowledge of a genetic predisposition affects a person's response to the disease and relationships with family members. For example, rheumatoid arthritis has a hereditary component. When a person develops the preliminary signs of any type of arthritis, his or her vision of the future will be quite different if a parent is severely handicapped by the disease than if no known family member has it.

A young man newly diagnosed with Friedreich's ataxia (a hereditary degenerative spinal disease) came to psychotherapy. The father was rejecting and quite abusive toward this son. Stricken by a crippling disease, the young man was struggling with his own reaction to an ultimately fatal disease and with his father's dysfunctional response. The psychotherapist was able to persuade the father to come to treatment with his son. Knowledge of the disease process and outcome served as a baseline, but learning that the disease was a recessive trait, partially inherited from the father, helped father and son understand and work through their problems (Thoene, 1995, pp. 272–273).

The environment may influence either the etiology or the severity of diseases (Griffith & Dambro, 1994, pp. 88–89). The incidence of black lung disease has decreased with changes in the mining industry. The incidence of asthma has increased dramatically, with the rise of environmental factors such as air pollution and overcrowded, insect-infested, urban housing. When people attribute their diseases to environmental causes (e.g., air, water, toxic waste dumps), accurately or not, they may become angry, especially if they believe their plight could have been prevented. Some people, however, feel more helpless or less inclined to take steps to alleviate their condition, on the assumption that the cause is external to them and they are powerless to change anything.

Some diseases are influenced by or associated with risk behaviors. AIDS is associated with unprotected sexual practices (although it may also be transmitted by other means, such as intravenous blood transfusions or from mother to fetus through the placenta). Lung cancer, emphysema, and heart disease are associated with smoking. Cirrhosis of the liver is associated with alcoholism. These diseases, too, may be caused by factors other than behavior, but they carry strong correlations with risk behaviors. The presence of diseases influenced by behavior often stirs guilt. People may stay in a posture of self-blame; they may move to a position of acceptance and "forgive" themselves; or they may flatly deny that their behavior is in any way related to their illness.

Diseases that occur as a part of the aging process create their own special psychological problems. They carry great uncertainty from day to day and definite certainty that the end of life is approaching. People who are facing multiple or overlapping physical problems are often concerned about what else can or will happen within a body that is no longer young. They worry about their decreasing abilities and increasing liabilities. Losses among the senses (e.g., sight, hearing, taste), in mobility, and in cognition and memory may take place. Susceptibility to disease and infection may increase. If the losses are great, it can be exceedingly difficult to face old age with courage and a sense of humor and to take pleasure in living.

Needs

The categories for the management of disease fall into four groups: auxiliary aids, mechanical or electrical; lifestyle changes;

medical treatment; and adjunctive treatment, including psycho-logical treatment. The availability of resources to manage disease does not necessarily mean that individuals will avail themselves of those options or even know that the options exist. Chapter 1 reported on the findings of a 2-year government study of super-vised cardiac rehabilitation programs that showed that fewer than one third of heart patients participated in these programs, although it was expected all could benefit (Leary, October 11, 1995). Numerous mechanical and electrical aids are available to assist people in daily living, such as eyeglasses, canes, hearing aids, braces, wheelchairs, jar openers, and handholds for tubs and showers. Some people welcome the availability of these aids, because they make life more comfortable and navigable. Others avoid their use, especially if the aid is visible, because they do not want to be viewed as handicapped in any way.

Lifestyle changes have been introduced in previous contexts, as in the cardiac rehabilitation programs and the diabetic regimen mentioned in the introduction to the templates. Lifestyle adjust-ments necessitated by disease, which are easy to list but difficult to implement and sustain, include changes in diet, exercise, sex-ual practices, and work. It may be necessary to change one's diet to low fat or no sugar, to reduced salt or limited calories, or per-haps to all of the above. Patients may need to increase, decrease, start, stop, or modify their exercise routines in some other way. They may need to alter their work patterns (e.g., to allow for dial-ysis). The construction worker who has lower extremity paralysis after a motor vehicle accident will need to find a different job. Some chronic fatigue syndrome patients have discovered that they must stop work altogether, because they do not have the energy to maintain sustained employment. Some of the changes affect only the individual, but others alter the lifestyle of family and partners significantly. Lifestyle issues are frequently a source of tension and contention in individuals, couples, and families.

Medical treatments include drugs, surgery, radiation therapy, and dialysis. Although these treatments can be life saving and contribute to an improved quality of life, they may cause effects in addition to the effects of the disease itself. Simple medications may be easily tolerated, but even aspirin can cause severe gastric problems if used frequently and in high doses. Powerful chemotherapy drugs, often used in rotating combinations among the different chemical agents, can overwhelm the patient with nausea, vomiting, and mouth sores. They can cause loss of hair (including eyelashes, which leaves the eyes unprotected). A teenager with cancer who was receiving both chemotherapy and radiation therapy described the taste of normally luscious foods as akin to "sucking on a lead pipe." Surgery can be relatively mild, as in the insertion of a shunt for renal dialysis, or it can be major, as in the removal of a colon or a uterus. Function may be improved postsurgery, as may happen following joint replacement for rheumatoid arthritis, or it may be worsened, as may happen following a colectomy for Crohn's disease. Radiation therapy may seem benign initially until the patient experiences debilitating fatigue or loses the sensation of taste. Late effects of irradiation (e.g., skin color changes, ovarian function failure) may emerge years after the treatment was administered.

Adjunctive treatments are often very beneficial, but some may be sought as panaceas for disease where none really exists. Physical therapy, occupational therapy, and psychotherapy are frequently used beneficial adjunctive therapies. These treatments aim to restore function where possible and help the patient cope with loss of function when necessary. Physical therapy helps the individual regain movement and enhances the strength and flexibility of the body. It may follow surgeries, such as hip or knee joint repairs and replacements. Physical therapy also can be used to facilitate function and to avoid or postpone surgery, as in treatment for spinal disk compression. It is an integral part of the treatment prescribed for rehabilitation after a stroke. Occupational therapy is designed to help patients better manage the activities of daily living in the kitchen, bathroom, or workroom. It can offer new skills, such as mastering a wheelchair or handling public transportation. Psychotherapy offers an array of services to patients with chronic illness. Chapter 5 is devoted entirely to such treatment and includes a menu of effective interventions.

Other adjunctive treatments can be therapeutic for people with chronic conditions. Acupuncture can be helpful to some patients for pain management. Aromatherapy (e.g., fragrantly scented baths) may be a "new age" trend that is little respected among professionals, but it is a source of comfort to many ill and distressed patients, and it does no harm. Yoga offers an alternative form of physical stretching, flexibility enhancement, and relaxation, which many patients find beneficial.

Considering all the management needs for a disease, one must decide whether the treatments will alter disease process or outcome. Many people do this kind of weighing and balancing intuitively or automatically: What will my life be like if I do use a hearing aid? What will happen to me if I do not stop smoking? What are the pros and cons of this medication or that surgery? Why do I keep reaching for salty oily snacks, when I'm already taking this medicine for my high cholesterol level? If I try this exercise, will I have more pain or less? Disease management can be onerous, but there are usually opportunities for improved adaptation and comfort.

The Threat Template

The Threat Template, an outgrowth of clinical observations in our medical and psychology practices, poses a different set of questions that provide another view of disease. These questions more closely address the psychological needs of a person living with chronic disease:

- Is the disease life threatening?
- Is the disease understood, but progressively disabling, not amenable to management?
- Is the disease not understood and unpredictable?
- Is the disease understood and manageable?

Perhaps more art than science in some respects, this approach to disease leads to the heart of the psychological reactions of patients and their families. Within a person and a family, anxiety is a concomitant for all the categories of the Threat Template, because each carries its own difficult challenges. Moreover, the answers to the questions in the Threat Template, when combined with those from the Medical Template, have implications that extend beyond the privacy of home, to the community and the culture.

Life Threatening

People become very frightened when disease poses a threat to life. Questions follow: "How soon?", "Can this be delayed?",

"Might there be a cure soon enough for me?" The element of time and the stages of dying take on significance. Being told that a disease will eventuate in death in 5 years is a different experience than being told the end will arrive soon. Nevertheless, to be informed of the cause of one's death and to be given a mathematical timetable for it is a profound subjective experience.

Consider the patient who has had repeated episodes of congestive heart failure, each one requiring mechanical ventilation and a week's stay in the hospital. Any episode may be the final one. How is the patient to live with this knowledge during the nonacute periods at home? One such patient we knew went to psychotherapy, because she felt the need to review her life and prepare to let go, and she was afraid of being alone during the final phase of her life. A widow whose children lived in another state, she did not have anyone else to help her to accomplish her goal. She wanted to die knowing that her life had been as good as it possibly could be under the circumstances; she needed a sense of integrity.

Progressive

Progressive diseases and conditions are those for which there are no cures and no known treatments to control decline, but that are not life threatening. It is a painful prospect to face life with a progressive disease over which one has little control. The presence of these diseases places people at risk for depression because of the associated losses and engendered helplessness. Hearing and vision losses with aging are examples of progressively disabling processes that may end in deafness and blindness.

Degenerative dementias such as Alzheimer's disease may be placed in this category because of their slow but insidious disease course. The etiology is not fully understood, but the disease process is clear, as is the outcome (Griffith & Dambro, 1994, pp. 24–25). Patients may live for many years with all body systems intact, except the mind. During the period that they still have partial or intermittent adequate cognitive function, they may have some awareness of the difficulties. When that happens, frustration and anxiety can become overwhelming. Ultimately, such individuals become totally incapacitated and need external care.

Unpredictable

There are many myths about the causes and cures for unpredictable diseases such as multiple sclerosis, rheumatoid arthritis, chronic fatigue syndrome, postviral syndrome, and post-Lyme syndrome. These diseases are not readily tolerated in our technological solution-focused society because of the aura of uncertainty that surrounds them. People with ambiguous diseases are often viewed as being depressed or psychosomatic, malingering, or using their symptoms for psychological secondary gain. Of course, any disease or symptom may be used for conscious or unconscious manipulation, but ambiguous diseases present an easier target for hostility or dismissal. If etiology is unknown and if symptoms do not remain fixed, how is one to understand such disease states?

A cautionary tale is in order. We know a woman with post-polio syndrome who struggled for several years with increasing disabilities. Physicians who did not understand the syndrome told her that her problems were "in her mind." Therefore, she refused to "give in" to her growing limitations. Refusing the use of crutches or a wheelchair, she crawled on the floor to move about her house. She was dismayed about her fatigue and her lower body weakness, atrophy, and pain, but she was determined to overcome her condition. Finally, her condition was evaluated by a knowledgeable physician who informed her about the late aftereffects of polio, which are believed to be caused by the breakdown of nerve cells damaged by the original bout with polio (Thoene, 1995, pp. 366–367). She was furious about the ignorance on the part of the previous physicians, but she was grateful to have new options, both medical and psychological. She purchased a wheelchair, moved her washer and dryer from the basement to the first floor of her home, and enrolled in a rehabilitation program. As a result of these changes, she was able to resume living with a disease process that is still poorly understood.

Manageable

Diseases are considered understood and manageable if treatment and appropriate lifestyle choices can control and mitigate the progression and impact on the body. By and large, the causes and effects of manageable diseases have been well described in the medical literature, and effective treatments are standardized and readily available. In the main, these are socially acceptable diseases and do not provoke undue anxiety in the general public (although the seriousness of a disease may be underestimated in the social consciousness). Diabetes and hypertension can be classified in this way, along with some skin cancers. Unlike the disease that carries with it a death threat, these are the diseases that give people more choices about their own lives.

Any disease that holds out the promise of choice also holds out the threat of despair. The unremitting quality of chronic disease exerts a demand on individuals to make the best choice every day in regard to food, exercise, stress reduction, medication, and rest. Under the press of illness, they may need help to make better, not always perfect, choices. Even manageable diseases can engender "battle fatigue" when individuals have to keep up the fight against disease and also face other demands or crises in life. Examples of adult patients with diabetes are given in chapters 4 and 5; children with diabetes are discussed in chapter 8.

Summary

Two templates have been introduced as a system by which psychotherapy practitioners who are not physicians may understand disease. The Medical Template frames the disease. One can use it to gain a basic understanding of any chronic illness. The Threat Template offers a continuum of danger placed by disease on a patient's existence. Diseases may change and developments may occur that would move a condition from one category to another. The categories themselves are not important as fixed assignments, but may point toward a shift in the pressing psychological and physical demands. The templates are meant to serve as a guide. They may be used in a general clinical practice as needed to gain and organize information relevant to psychological treatment for chronic disease. Worksheets for the four templates are included on pages 215–218.

3

The Response Template: A View of the Patient's Search for Help

Psychological reactions and coping responses stimulated by the arrival and endurance of a chronic illness can be described in many ways. In devising a new set of categories for the Response Template, we think it is more accurate from a clinical standpoint (as well as experience-near) to present a typical progression of psychological events in a chronic disease process.

The adaptation to a disease process is a journey, with recognizable markers along the way. Problems may occur at any of the crossroads during the journey. Holland and Rowland (1989) reviewed adaptation to illness across the life span and described five common problem sources, which they labeled the "five D's": distance in interpersonal relations, dependence versus independence, disability disruptions to achievement, disfigurement (impairments to body image and integrity), and death fears or anxieties. These kinds of disruptions are expected, although the salience of each changes according to individual circumstances. Difficulty in any of the five areas may occur during any of the stages of the response sequence described below.

In this chapter, the focus is on the response process, not on disease per se. We hope it will be helpful to clinicians in identifying where individual patients may be in their responses to an illness and, thus, used in conjunction with the templates presented in the previous chapter. Taken together, the templates give a holographic view for understanding the patient with a chronic illness and for setting the context for the development of a meaningful psychological treatment plan.

Response Sequence and Influences

A typical pattern develops in response to an illness that becomes chronic. The pattern seems to follow a characteristic sequence.

The Response Template
□ Initial response: Something is wrong.
□ Awareness of chronicity: Something continues to be wrong.
□ Disorganization: Whatever is wrong is disturbing my life in significant ways.
□ Intensified wish for a cure: Whatever is wrong must be changed.
□ Acknowledgment of helplessness: I cannot change what is wrong.
□ Adaptation to illness: How can I live with what is wrong and is changing my life?

The Response Template is a continuum. Patients begin with an awareness that something is wrong. With time, the disruption of their lives in some manner causes various levels of disorganization in their usual ways of coping with existence. Eventually, they attempt to reestablish the previous order of life or to reorganize to cope in some way with the problems caused by the illness.

A number of factors influence the sequence, such as mode of onset, disease characteristics, coping style, special characteristics, and stage of life. In particular, the mode of onset of a chronic illness has a marked effect on the response to the intrusion of disease. The onset may be an abrupt event that catapults the patient into a radical change immediately, such as a sudden myocardial infarction (heart attack) or a spinal cord injury that causes immediate paralysis. The onset may be gradual and make itself felt as a more insidious process, such as diabetes or hypertension. The onset may be episodic or intermittent, with acute flare-ups and periods of quiescence. Examples of diseases with intermittent modes are asthma, rheumatoid arthritis, and chronic fatigue syndrome.

Response to illness is influenced by the disease characteristics themselves, as discussed in chapter 2. (See the Medical Template for influential factors such as expected outcome and management needs.) The coping style and adaptive capacities of an individual also have a strong effect on the response to illness. These matters of enduring personality organization and level of function are discussed in detail in chapter 4.

Some special characteristics of a disease may significantly alter the response to illness: disease visibility, the level of social acceptance (vs. stigma) associated with the disease, and severity of threat to life. For the most part, it is harder to bear a visible disease or condition than a nonvisible one. Visible signs of neurofibromatosis (a disorder characterized by brown skin spots and bone and tissue deformities), cystic acne, or a limb amputation, for example, often produce a wish to hide and a self-protecting withdrawal. The removal of a breast or testicular tumor leaves a visible aftermath of scarring. Although the scars are not in public view, they may exert a similar wish to withdraw from intimate relationships. Nonvisible diseases allow the patient wider latitude in deciding whether to reveal their presence. They may also make it possible for patients to ignore and deny the disease, to the detriment of their health and well-being.

Some diseases are horrifying to patients and their families because of the social impact and associated stigma. Patients with diseases such as AIDS, tuberculosis, and leprosy are often shunned in society. Myths about the diseases and those who suffer from them often evoke rejection of the patients as a source of contagion or as bad or immoral persons.

When disease poses a threat to life, the entire sequential process may be speeded up. People whose lives hinge on receiving an organ transplant or on an experimental new chemotherapy protocol may be so overwhelmed by death anxiety that they cycle rapidly through disorganization, wishes, and helplessness in an attempt to master the experience.

The stage of life at which the disease occurs poses special problems that affect the response to illness because of the potential interference to the accomplishment of the stage tasks. Erikson's (1963) widely used descriptors of life stage tasks may be used as a summary list of psychological function areas that may be adversely affected: trust (infancy), autonomy (toddlerhood), initiative (preschool), industry (latency), identity (adolescence), intimacy (young adulthood), generativity (middle adulthood), and integrity (older adulthood). A sick infant is totally dependent on adults for medical care, pain relief, and reassurance. A teenager's response to illness will interact with the concerns of the age (e.g., "Can I be like the other kids in my crowd?" "Can I get my driver's license?"). A 42-year-old bread-winner, at the height of power and responsibility at home and at work, may be ill prepared to let go of that power and face illness. Elderly individuals with chronic illnesses are often concerned about resources for their care, the loss of autonomy, and often the loss of the ability to live at home.

The Initial Response: Something Is Wrong

When people get acutely sick, they respond initially in their customary ways. They go to their doctor, or take to bed, or self-medicate, or attempt to ignore the illness, or seek soothing or caretaking from others, or minimize or maximize the process. They also attempt to understand what is happening to them (e.g., "It must be the virus that's going around"). Some people do not experience themselves as ill, however. Instead, they may have one initial symptom, like neck pain, which may be attributed to sleeping in an awkward position; or muscle weakness in the legs, attributed to too much or too little exercise; or fatigue, attributed to generic "stress." Some people have a single specific symptom, such as thirst or a "lump." People organize information in ways they find helpful in order to make sense of what is happening to them and to avoid anxiety.

The mode of onset often determines the initial response. The response to abrupt spinal cord injury is usually shock, both physiologically and psychologically. The person may not be able to fathom the extent and implications of the injury immediately, but he or she does get immediate medical attention. An abrupt heart attack heralds the presence of coronary artery disease. Most people seek immediate help, but some deny progressive symptoms (e.g., "it's only heartburn") until they are over-whelmed by crushing chest pain.

With a gradual and insidious onset, the response to disease is likely to be affected by the person's ability to self-explain symptoms and by any tendencies to minimize or maximize symptoms.

The severity of symptoms also affects the response. The onset of diabetes produces excessive thirst, fatigue, and weight loss. Colon cancer produces weight loss as well as changes in stool character and color. People with either condition often wait to seek medical attention until their own attempts at accounting for what is wrong no longer suffice.

In disease states that are intermittent in nature, there may be a long span of time between episodes. People who have asthma or rheumatoid arthritis may minimize and postpone seeking medical attention for years. Sometimes a person may tumble into an acute crisis episode and seek help. A person might go to a local hospital emergency room for relief from the respiratory distress of an asthma attack while still denying the presence of underlying disease.

Awareness of Chronicity: Something Continues to Be Wrong

Symptoms may diminish or abate temporarily, may worsen, may shift from one body site to another, or may stay the same. Patients may receive a tentative diagnosis, a series of conflicting diagnoses, or a definite diagnosis. They may continue to seek medical help or may withdraw, hoping to heal naturally. When they do not recover, frustration escalates. Their anxiety levels rise, and they may start to speculate about death, incapacitation, pain, abandonment, or spreading the disease to others. Frightening or anxiety-provoking fantasies may be conscious or unconscious. For example, some people may errect a wall of denial to cope with their fears but not aware that they are using a defensive strategy.

If the onset of the problem has been abrupt, as in patients with spinal cord injury and myocardial infarction, the awareness of chronicity happens quickly. It may happen instantly, or it may take place over a week's time, as the person makes the transition from acute experience to assimilation of the implications for chronicity. The realization that the severe disability will not resolve can and does generate high levels of anxiety and a profound grief reaction.

Ambiguous waxing and waning diseases may go on for years before the person comes to grips with the chronicity. At the outset of a medical evaluation, the physician is unable to provide certainty. Typically, the patient receives mixed responses, based on an inconclusive history and physical and laboratory findings. More tests (e.g., biopsies, X-ray studies) are recommended. Return visits are recommended. Consultation with another physician may be suggested. Both the patient and the doctor may have unanswered questions about diagnosis, treatment, cure, and the veracity of the symptoms. Often, multiple laboratory tests give inconclusive results. For example, until very recently, diagnosis of the typical patient with multiple sclerosis took 6 months to a year. Some of the diseases to be "ruled out" are likely to be serious. Therefore, the patient's concern about his or her health and safety naturally intensifies, when the fantasies about the presence of a possible life-debilitating or life-threatening disease begin to develop.

When the medical establishment is unable to reach a definitive physical diagnosis and finds no clear cause for the patient's suffering, the responses of other people often are negative or become negative with time. The patient's physicians, family, employers, co-workers, and friends tire of the complaints and of the inability to carry on normally. They may begin to treat the patient as a malingerer, a selfish attention-seeker, or a "crazy" person. In some cases, they doubt that the patient is really and legitimately ill in a socially acceptable sense. Many of these characterizations are manifestations of hostility, anxiety, and frustration, engendered by the ambiguity of such an unpredictable and unresolving situation. Examples of ambiguous disease processes that trigger doubt and hostility in many people's minds are multiple sclerosis, post-Lyme and postviral syndromes, and chronic fatigue syndrome. Patients with illnesses characterized by society as marginal or psychosomatic may be forced into the position of denying the psychological stress taking place within them. They must then split off the rejected psychological contribution to the total experience of illness. They insist on the truth of a "real" physical illness and reject categorically any psychological components whatsoever. This splitting process reflects the mind–body split held by Western culture in general and by modern medicine to a large degree, so it is not a surprising reaction.

Disorganization: Whatever Is Wrong Is Disturbing
My Life In Significant Ways

The continuing presence of disease forces change on the patients' life functions and usual routines. Symptoms are often a major impediment to quality of life. Patients, families, and employers can no longer rely on the patient. Patients may not be able to continue their jobs or education, or they may need to scale back hours or predictability of hours. Family roles and responsibilities may be eliminated, reduced, or altered. Symptoms, disease, and the surrounding anxiety are often tiring in and of themselves, but the difficulty may be magnified by their interference with the ability to rest or sleep. Tired and sick people are apt to lose their sense of humor, as well as their spirit and energy for play.

Persistent disability may cause the patient great discouragement. For example, the necessity of managing constant chronic pain takes a toll, until and unless the pain can be relieved sufficiently. The chronicity of disease may be lessened at times, which allows people needed hope. Sometimes, the lessening takes the form of a remission and eventually a cure. Often, however, the remission does not last, and the resurgence or recurrence of disease is a frightening and devastating blow. Physical disability that is erratic and unpredictable is a maddening and frustrating experience.

When disease and disability persist, a true psychological disorganization begins, especially in the face of an uncertain future course or timetable. Signs of disorganization that may reflect deeper processes include, but are not limited to, scattered thinking, intrusive thoughts, volatile shifts in affect, persistent anxiety, and withdrawn self-absorption. In general, most people seem to focus only on the specific symptoms of distress and do not recognize that an underlying disorganization process is taking place.

To handle the potential threat to the self, the patient seeks psychological reassurance from a network of physicians, family, colleagues, friends, and maybe even a psychotherapist. With time, anxiety and fear spread in the patient's emotional landscape. Some patients also become angry quite early on, a response that is influenced by the individual's tolerance for frustration or propensity to blame the external world for internal states, or that occurs when their sense of entitlement is thwarted. Some patients cover anxiety with anger. However, almost everyone faced with serious frustration eventually becomes angry at the unfairness of the situation. It is a natural response, but it may require assistance to anticipate, manage, and work through. Some patients are unable to handle their anger, but no one notices until they explode, and only then are they referred for psychotherapy.

Patients' negative internal messages go hand in hand with the messages from the outside world. The responses of other people have an extraordinary impact at this vulnerable psychological crossroads in their inner life experience. Patients' losses are growing. They face the internal loss of a familiar sense of self, function, and identity, and they may be faced with the external loss of support or contact with important other people at work, in the social milieu, or even among family members. For most patients, financial losses, caused by diminished income and increased medical expenses, are also significant. In response to these and other losses, a tendency toward withdrawal, isolation, and depressive signs develops.

Patients' psychological distress constellation may include a hypersensitive self-absorption with the body, anxiety and confusion about what "really" is happening or will happen, frustration with the lack of control over events, anger at others for not helping matters, guilt over causing the illness or about taking up the time and resources of others, self-doubt about managing the experienced illness, self-pity over one's poor lot, and depression surrounding the hopeless and helpless elements within the self. All of these symptoms both reflect and push the underlying process that has been referred to previously as *psychological disorganization*.

At this point, some people give up and retire from life, entrenched in their sick or lost position, but for most people the attempt to cope continues. Patients try to stave off disorganization and to retain a stable sense of self. Too often, out of necessity, patients develop a compensatory reaction formation against a deteriorating inner psychological compass and deny the importance of their emotional responses. Instead, they focus only on their physical states. Most people struggle courageously to reorganize themselves internally, without conscious awareness of the process or assistance that would help them to navigate the disorganizing transition period.

Intensified Wish for a Cure: Whatever Is Wrong Must Be Changed

The search for assistance expands in many directions. Patients may seek help through consultation at the nation's major medical diagnostic centers. They may locate groups of people with the same disease, learning from them about the disease and acquiring tips about how to manage it or where to seek further help. If medical consultation does not yield promising results, they may select strategies from among many alternative body therapies and palliatives such as nutritional regimens, acupuncture, massage, and exercise. They may embark on a religious or philosophical quest for solace, cure, or meaning in the effort to understand and to withstand the physical disease and the emotional disorganization. Their search process uses great stores of inner resources.

The focus of patients and their most important wish is for a return to the premorbid physical, psychological, and functional self. The strength of the wish to return to the "normal" or "old" self seems to grow in proportion to the strength of the disorganizing challenge to the identity. Magical thinking processes and superstitious beliefs are typical as the threat to the self continues from within and without. For example, patients may feel guilty for being ill. They may believe that the illness is a punishment for misdeeds or poor habits or may imagine that the problem lies in not trying hard enough because of laziness or lack of moral fiber, grit, and determination. At the other extreme, patients may blame themselves for working too hard, having Type A personalities, or overdoing exercise. A tendency to minimize one's role in illness or to maximize it to the point of believing one can control the illness may be incorporated into the individual's magical thinking process. Magical thinking is often a by-product of the wish for a cure that cannot be satisfied.

The wish for a cure may be present throughout the entire response to illness. This powerful wish to be freed, saved, released, or healed, no matter how it is expressed, grows exponentially with an increase in the life-threatening nature of the disease. A person may start the response process with such a wish when illness is very grave, painful, or incapacitating. On the other hand, this stage in the process may be less obvious and pressing in a person who is able to reach an easier adaptation with a less intrusive disease.

Acknowledgment of Helplessness: I Cannot Change What Is Wrong

Neither the disease nor the psychological process is linear. It is important to understand the high frustration of the entire experience. Patients have tremendous difficulty adapting to the persistent course, to debilitating symptoms that are variable or unrelenting, to the reactions of others, to the loss of role function, and to the psychological symptoms of disorganization. Patients will have good days and bad days, setbacks, and sometimes even periods of relative well-being. Nevertheless, searches for new treatments will have failed to halt the disease and the psychological disorganization. Ultimately, the losses involved must be acknowledged and faced: Life will never be the same again. As this occurs, a healthy grief, or perhaps a profound depression, develops.

This is the phase in the response process where patients fully recognize their helplessness to change what is wrong. Acknowledging helplessness does not mean that patients give up any of the adaptive responses that help manage or regulate the illness. It does not mean they abandon faith, in either the spiritual sense or the personal sense of efficacy that is focused on living as meaningful and satisfying a life as is possible. It simply means not trying to undo what has already occurred and cannot be undone. When patients relinquish a fruitless strategy, there is usually room in their internal worlds to face the losses of the past and the fears about the future.

Adaptation to Chronic Illness: How Can I Live With What Is Wrong and Is Changing My Life?

Patients respond differently to disease, disorganization, and helplessness, depending on their capacity for creative adaptation in their lives, the severity of the illness, and the support available in their environment. They are challenged to find coping strategies as the disease process changes and as they are changed by it.

Coping strategies are successful only to the extent that they are congruent with patients' normative personality style and level of functioning.

Patients also differ in the degrees of help needed to reorganize within their altered realities. They may seek psychological help spontaneously, or they may be referred for psychological help. They may struggle to reorganize on their own. They may not reorganize and refuse help. Some are at risk for suicide. Patients whose diseases have special characteristics (e.g., visibility or stigma) often find the task of adaptation more difficult. In such instances, patients not only must cope with the disease but also must find a way to deal with the reactions of others.

Despite serious obstacles, many patients are able to develop a restructuring of their lives and internal sense of stability. They are able to reorganize in a healthy way. A few are so brittle they do not adapt; instead, they collapse psychologically. Some have an encapsulated neurotic adaptation with a limited range of possibilities; they become subsumed into the patient role or are viewed as society's discards or cranks. Some are transformed, like the phoenix rising from the ashes, and show significant gains as they reorganize their lives. Most patients need support and assistance at some point in their process of reorganization. This is true even for patients who reconsolidate in their acceptance of permanent disability or impending death. It is necessary for psychotherapists to understand the continuum of disorganization and reorganization, as well as to make use of usual diagnostic and clinical skills, if they want to understand their patients' experiential journey through life with an illness.

Michael: Case Illustration of a Patient's Response to Illness

The following case example is limited to material relevant to the patient's response to illness. We have excluded comment or analysis on the professional controversy surrounding the disease and on the personality structure of the patient in order to keep the focus on the narrative line that follows his experience and world view.

Initial Response: Something Is Wrong

Michael was a 42-year-old professor of music theory in a large university. His promising career was on the rise, and he had a new book that was about to be published. He was a divorced father of two adolescent children who lived with their mother during the week and spent weekends with him. He was involved in a relatively new relationship with Beth, which he expected to lead to marriage. He was a nonsmoker, rarely drank alcohol, and had never used street drugs.

For several months Michael felt more tired than usual. On three occasions he took his children back to their mother earlier than planned; once he was too tired to take them at all and canceled his scheduled weekend visitation. Over the next 6 months, he had three episodes of acute pharyngitis (a sore throat), and each time he sought medical advice and received antibiotics. Michael's physician documented fever, swollen glands, and recurrent streptococcus infection.

Awareness of Chronicity: Something Continues to Be Wrong

Michael became increasingly fatigued. He slept 10 to 12 hours a day. He stopped writing. Visits with his children became more infrequent. His social life with Beth was reduced to simple meals in a local restaurant and occasional movies on videotape at home. As the fatigue continued and new infections occurred, Michael again sought a consultation with his physician. He knew something was wrong with his body. The medical work-up included blood tests, which were all within normal limits. There was no evidence of diabetes, anemia, or Lyme disease. A stress test was normal, although Michael complained of fatigue during the test. The physician had no answers for him.

Disorganization: Whatever Is Wrong Is Disturbing My Life in Significant Ways

At the end of the first year of illness, Michael was frankly worried that something was very wrong with him. His fatigue became so debilitating that he requested a reduction in his teaching hours, which was granted by his department. The reduction relieved his daily activity burden somewhat, but it was financially constraining and increased his anxiety further. He was discouraged and slipped into a self-berating mode: "What's wrong with me? Why can't I get things together?" The recurrent sore throats and swollen glands persisted. The physician prescribed a course of antidepressant medication, which Michael was willing to try.

Michael's sons and former wife became frustrated with the many aborted weekend visits. They believed he was malingering and was shirking his responsibilities. Beth was patient with him, but she was worried about his health. Michael returned to the psychotherapist he had consulted at the time of his divorce. The therapist thought Michael was depressed and was frustrated by his poor response to psychotherapy, his increasing fatigue, and his decreasing job and social functioning.

Intensified Wish for a Cure: Whatever Is Wrong Must Be Changed

At this point Michael's life had become so disrupted by fatigue and recurrent infections that he decided to arrange a specialist consultation and evaluation at a major medical diagnostic and treatment center. He was determined to find a cure. There, after many more tests, Michael was informed that he had chronic fatigue syndrome. He was told that the cause, course, and outcome could be neither established nor predicted, but the fatigue and the recurrent infections could be expected to continue. He returned home, discouraged.

As time passed, Michael was barely able to keep up with the reduced teaching schedule. His physician suggested he take a disability leave from work, for a period of time. The leave entailed a further loss of income. Michael worried that his life would continue its downward spiral unless he could find someone, somewhere, who really understood his disease. He redoubled his efforts to find help. He spent money he could ill afford to travel to Boston and New York for consultations with specialists on chronic fatigue syndrome. He also tried herbal cures and gamma globulin injections. He changed to a different antidepressant medication. He worked with his psychotherapist, who continued to feel helpless and who encouraged Michael to seek new alternative forms of help. She, too, was struggling, along with Michael, to change what was wrong. She unintentionally colluded with his intensified wish for a cure.

By the time Michael turned 44, his life as he had known it was gone. His promising career as a music professor was lost. His sons had tried to understand their father's fatigue, but they felt abandoned by him. They were sure that if he just tried a little harder, he could get well. Beth had come to believe there was no future for her in a relationship with Michael, and she left him.

Acknowledgment of Helplessness: I Cannot Change What Is Wrong

Michael felt hopeless. He began to review his losses and to talk about them. His physician moved away from the area, and he had to choose a new one. The new physician reviewed all of Michael's records, including his extensive evaluations from the Boston and New York centers. Then she met with him and listened to him. Instead of dismissing his complaints or offering the promise of cures, she suggested that he might always have some degree of fatigue. In addition, she asked for a consultation with Michael and his psychotherapist.

The three-way consultation was productive. When the therapist realized the disease was probably going to be incapacitating to Michael, possibly for years to come, she stopped supporting his intensified wish for a cure. She began to help Michael work through his losses, his fears about his future, and his guilty sense that he must be responsible for all that had happened to him (if only he had not worked so intensely in the year prior to illness; if only he had done something sooner; if only he would try harder; and so forth).

Adaptation to Illness: How Can I Live With What Is Wrong and Is Changing My Life?

As Michael acknowledged the helplessness he felt (but had been covering), he began to experience some relief. His sleep slowly began to improve. He began a very minimal exercise program, stretching for 5 minutes a day. Gradually, he increased his exercise time and started walking for a few minutes every day. He realized that a return to his former schedule of teaching and writing would not be possible. Instead, he began a light schedule of teaching private piano students in his home, two students a day, four afternoons a week.

He still experienced episodic infections that would necessitate his canceling the student appointments and ending the exercise program. He struggled with depressive reactions in response to these return bouts of worsened fatigue and illness. Yet as each episode ended, he resumed his teaching and exercise. It was frustrating for him to start over again, walking only a few minutes a day. As Michael learned to live with his disease, his sons began to respect his perseverance. One of the boys spent increased amounts of time with him, as his own schedule of activities permitted, and the renewal of their relationship was very gratifying to Michael.

Today, Michael still longs for a cure for his disease, or at least a remission that is more substantial than his present circumstance, but he no longer spends his limited resources of energy and money trying to cure chronic fatigue syndrome. He does read regularly about his condition, and both he and his physician watch for news that may bring further improvement or a cure. For now, the teaching, a bit of writing, and minimal but regular exercise use the energy he had spent on a frantic search for the cure for his disease. He is tentatively expanding his social life. He continues to work on his issues of loss, fear, and guilt, whenever they resurface. Michael's illness journey is not yet finished, but he has achieved a reconsolidation and has been able to move ahead. He has successfully reorganized his life in response to his illness.

Summary

The Response Template is a view of the typical sequence of responses to chronic illness experienced by patients. The case of Michael illustrates this continuum of responses. The therapist in Michael's case became much more effective when she became aware of the disease outcome, process, etiology, and needs (the Medical Template). As she understood the level of threat to Michael's way of life (the Threat Template) and realized the helplessness he was experiencing in response to the illness (the Response Template), she was able to help him move on to better adaptation to the disease.

4

The Psychological Template: The Personality Dimension

Psychological intervention is more likely to be successful when the clinician understands the premorbid personality structure of the chronically ill person. The press of illness may be so great that even an exceptionally well adjusted person with good emotional resilience is threatened with psychological disorganization. However, anecdotal evidence suggests that patients with a preexisting disturbance or deficit in psychological functioning are even more likely to require the services of psychotherapists when the burden of physical illness strains their resources beyond personal tolerances. Therefore, diagnosis of both level and style of organization becomes paramount. In this chapter, we introduce clinical examples of personality differences first, followed by the Psychological Template for the evaluation of personality styles in response to the stressor of disease. Just as we gave a frame for understanding disease with the Medical Template, this fourth template gives a framework for understanding personality and constitutes an essential element in the hologram of the person who is ill.

For the Psychological Template, five specific categories of functioning are considered in assessing personality style. It becomes increasingly important to understand how the patient manages the reciprocal impact and influence of the Psychological Template areas as a part of the response to disease.

The Psychological Template
- ☐ Reality
- ☐ Anxiety
- ☐ Relationships
- ☐ Cognition
- ☐ Mastery–Competence

Diabetes as Experienced by Four Individuals

Whether and how individuals restructure and reorganize internal experience in response to chronic physical illness is dependent largely on their enduring personality structure. To illustrate the variety of response capabilities, four patients with diabetes are presented. Although the disease is the same in each instance, the patients are very different; all of them suffer from anxiety, but their strengths and weaknesses affect the ways in which they are capable of responding to the disease and living their lives. In treating each of them, it was necessary to understand the characteristic ways in which each dealt with the disease. (Note: The psychological treatment summaries for these patients are presented in the next chapter. Only personality structure is discussed throughout the remainder of this chapter.)

Denise

At the onset of diabetes, Denise was a 40-year-old woman who was 100 pounds overweight. Her mother, her four sisters, and her daughter were chronically obese and also had diabetes. The mother had heart failure and was on renal dialysis for kidney failure. One sister was also on dialysis. The family used food to soothe themselves and each other. Food was associated with affection and attachment, and it was used to smother emptiness and anxiety.

Denise was the first in her family to complete high school. She was employed as a food service worker for a large institution and had held the job for 10 years. She lived with her adult daughter and served as a caretaker for her family and friends.

Over the course of her life, she had intermittent relationships with men; however, none involved sustained intimacy. She had many women friends from her church, whom she saw regularly and with whom she occasionally went on vacations.

During the initial physician evaluation, Denise appeared competent and seemed successful by her own and her family's standards. Nevertheless, she responded to the anxiety generated by the diagnosis of diabetes with increased eating. She told her physician and others that her disease was "just a touch" of diabetes, and she took on a second job as a waitress, ostensibly for the extra income. She reasoned that she was fine, because she felt well and had no difficulty with her increased work hours.

Denise was likeable, and she attempted to please those involved in her health care. A cyclical pattern began to emerge. Under the physician's guidance, she would lose 5 or 10 pounds and feel proud of her achievement. Then she would experience an emotional upset in one of her relationships (her lover would not arrive as planned, her daughter would stay out overnight, her sister would not speak to her), and the overeating would resume. Denise would regain the lost weight and gain additional weight as well.

Denise was a "concrete thinker." Her physician had been discussing diets for her that were based on food exchanges, and he had assumed that she understood, because she faithfully wrote down everything she ate. However, Denise was unable to grasp the principles of food exchange. For example, she eliminated fried chicken from her diet, but substituted fried shrimp instead, not understanding their parity of saturated fat content. Her literal cognitive style led to serious problems in managing insulin dosages as the disease progressed.

Denise's diabetic condition worsened and her erratic eating increased. During this time her mother died, and Denise gained another 50 pounds. She developed the initial signs of kidney failure and heart failure. Nevertheless, she minimized her worsening condition, attributing it to "stress" and "grief." She continued employment at her two jobs, but there were periods of time when she was unable to work because of her heart condition and the need to regulate her insulin. Shortly thereafter, Denise's sister died of renal failure.

As Denise's condition worsened, her physician recommended renal dialysis as treatment for her own failing kidneys. The physician informed her that she had a favorable prognosis with the treatment, unlike her mother and sister. Denise refused adamantly. She believed that the renal dialysis had caused the deaths of her mother and sister. She did not believe that dialysis could substantially prolong her own life. At that point, the physician recommended psychological evaluation, and Denise agreed to talk with a psychologist.

Richard

Richard was an intelligent 35-year-old man with a PhD in chemistry. He was 40 pounds overweight when initially diagnosed with insulin-dependent diabetes, although he had actually lost weight in the month prior to diagnosis because of the disease. He was single but had been living with a woman for the past 3 years in a committed relationship. They had marriage plans and were hoping to start a family.

As a rational scientist, Richard functioned in an obsessive–compulsive style. When he became ill and was told that he had diabetes and would need insulin, he used his compulsivity to defend against the anxiety he could not allow himself to feel directly. In 1 year he lost 60 pounds. He exercised 1 to 2 hours a day and worked 10 to 12 hours a day. He consulted the most renowned diabetologists in the country and was controlling his insulin requirements to a level of only two to three units daily.

As time passed, Richard became increasingly preoccupied with illness. He went to the emergency room of his local hospital in the middle of the night on several occasions with colds. He was afraid of becoming more sick and of his diabetes getting out of control. Richard managed to maintain his rigorous work schedule, but his obsessions and compulsions about his health, diet, and exercise left less and less time for relaxation or for relationships. He began to suffer from insomnia associated with intrusive thoughts of physical illness. Finally, his fiancée broke off the relationship and moved out of their shared house. With that loss as the precipitating event, Richard, whose diabetes was under near-perfect control, sought psychotherapy.

Marion

Marion was 45 years old when her physician told her that she had diabetes. She worked as an accountant in a job she had trained for 8 years earlier. She was married and had an adolescent daughter. The physician thought she had a stable life, although her history revealed both mental and physical abuse by her husband. She had received psychotherapy in the past and had decided to remain in her marriage, despite its problems. Also notable in her history at the time was the death of her mother 2 years earlier from complications of diabetes. With the onset of diabetes, Marion set herself the task of controlling her blood sugar and weight.

Marion did well for the first few months. She lost 20 pounds and kept meticulous charts of her daily blood sugars, exercise, and weight. Her blood sugars returned to normal, and she felt sure that with continued control she would be able to manage her chronic illness.

One day Marion came into her physician's office, wringing her hands, upset, and reporting that she was not eating properly or exercising. She described herself as "bad," but said she felt overwhelmed and did not feel up to following her regimen. The physician supported her and Marion was able to reestablish her program. She did well again for another 4 months or so. Then, once again she presented herself in her physician's office, wringing her hands and berating herself for her failure, despite improved and more rigid record keeping.

After several relapses, the physician realized that despite very compulsive patterns of monitoring her own behavior, Marion was not coping. Instead, she was lapsing into "near depression" with her repeated episodes of self-deprecation. The physician suggested Marion return for psychotherapy, which she did.

Judy

Judy was a 64-year-old homemaker with a 30-year history of diabetes, on insulin for 20 of those years, when she transferred to the care of a new physician because of a change in health insurance. She had raised four children, all of whom were married. She had six grandchildren, ages 2 to 12, whom she tended regularly. She worried about the problems of her children, but otherwise seemed to her physician to be content with life.

In managing her diabetes, Judy kept copious but erratic blood sugar records, and this puzzled her physician. Sometimes, she would record the early morning and late afternoon results as he requested. Often, she would record blood sugar checks at 3:30 A.M. or 4:30 A.M., as well as five or six scattered times throughout a day. She explained the varied testing times by expressing her belief that stress altered her blood sugars. Furthermore, she also adjusted her insulin according to anticipated stress by taking extra units if she expected to be "stressed" on a given day. The irregular insulin dosages caused several episodes of hypoglycemia, necessitating hospitalization.

The physician attempted to help Judy reestablish a regular pattern of insulin use by seeing her quite frequently, almost weekly. Despite this intensive response to her, she continued the prolific blood sugar testing and recording at all hours. One day, when Judy appeared to be disoriented and confused, the physician hospitalized her for a complete medical workup. There were no significant findings, and her blood sugars remained normal throughout the several days of hospitalization. On discharge, the physician referred her to a psychologist for a consultation.

Denise, Richard, Marion, and Judy responded to diabetes in ways that were characteristic for them. The valence of attitudes and behaviors they had toward their disease and its management were typical of the attitudes and behaviors they used in adapting to other inner and outer forces impinging on their lives. Each person worked to minimize the tensions and anxiety brought on by the pressures of the disease and its unremitting management needs.

Personality Structures

There are many different and overlapping systems for understanding an individual's characteristic pattern of response to stress. Psychodynamically oriented practitioners are educated to think of personality organization according to type of personality (e.g., hysterical, obsessive–compulsive, paranoid, depressive, schizoid, narcissistic), which takes into account structure, defenses, psychopathology, and adaptation style. Drive, ego, object relations, and self theory elements all contribute to an understanding of the complexity of human personality.

The salient features of personality theory selected for the assessment of the person with chronic illness are personality type (enduring constellation of organization), mental and functional capacities (high to low, availability and workability of defenses), key trait factors (positive to negative scale), ego functions (identification of strengths and deficits), and personal hierarchies (the uniqueness of a person). All help us to better select the kinds of interventions that our patients can hear and use. The following brief examples from the literature highlight the theoretical underpinnings for these features.

Psychoanalytic Diagnosis: Understanding Personality Structure in the Clinical Process by Nancy McWilliams (1994) provides a complete and accessible discussion on character structure. In the section "Character, Character Pathology, and Situational Factors," she noted: "Assessment of someone's character structure, even in the absence of a personality disorder, gives the therapist an idea of what kinds of interventions will be assimilable by the client and what style of relatedness will make him or her most receptive to efforts to help" (p. 147). She distinguished dynamics from pathology and character from responsivity, which we find to be particularly useful distinctions in the treatment of patients for whom physical illness must be factored into the clinical picture.

Along with character types, one may classify personality according to functional capacities and mental functioning. Kernberg (1976) evaluated a range of character states that includes material related to instinctual development, ego and defenses, superego, affects, object relations, and interpersonal relationships. His system assesses each category of functioning and capacity from low to high, psychotic to normal. In her seminal article, "The So-Called Good Hysteric," Zetzel (1968) presented a schema that differentiates treatment outcome for hysterically organized patients according to four levels of functioning (heretofore, hysterical personalities were assumed to be on a high level of neuroticism). McWilliams (1994) highlighted the importance of a conceptual grid, with level of functioning on one axis and type of personality on the other.

Stone (1993) has proposed an integration of the five-factor models of personality. Those models derive their name from the irreducible number of personality dimensions (culled from hundreds of positive and negative traits) identified by personality researchers. Stone used the widely used factor terms of McCrae and John (1992): extraversion, agreeableness, conscientiousness, neuroticism, and openness. He examined the relationship between the superfactors and personality disorders in a heuristic attempt to develop a unified model for the understanding of abnormalities in personality. His approach offers another step toward understanding treatment possibilities and impediments.

Based on work by Bellak and Small (1977), Small (1979) noted the importance of assessing ego functions, because one or more ego functions are affected in every emotional disturbance. These clinical researchers suggested that treatment interventions be specifically tailored to address problems in any of the functions, which are defined as reality testing; judgment; sense of reality; regulation and control of drives, affects, and impulses; object relations; thought processes; adaptive regression in the service of the ego; defensive functions; stimuli barrier; autonomous functions; synthetic–integrative function; and mastery–competence. Within the construct of ego, people draw on their individual ego resources to mediate experience and create meaning for themselves. Problems in any of the 12 functions adversely affect a person's ability to handle the effects and consequences of illness; conversely, serious physical illness may have a temporary or permanent adverse effect on some functions of the ego.

Pine (1991) has contributed the concept of hierarchies and fluidity to our understanding of personality. He observed that "the phenomenon of urge, of adaptation, of object relations and of self are all reflected in anything the person does" (p. 115). Sets of issues become organizing for a person; the organizations of sets of issues constitute personal hierarchies. Pine stipulated that "there is no substitute for evaluation and understanding of individual history and individual function" (p. 115).

Psychological Template

The Psychological Template, a set of questions for thinking about personality, is a guide for evaluating and understanding the characteristic ways in which a person responds to significant stress. Our theoretical underpinning is psychoanalytic; however, the template questions are designed for the clinical utility of practitioners from varying disciplines and orientations. Practitioners from orientations other than the psychoanalytic may wish to add to or reframe the questions for use within other theoretical systems.

The five questions are as follows:

- How does the person manage reality?
- How does the person manage anxiety?
- How does the person manage relationships?
- How does the person manage cognition?
- What is the person's mastery–competence level?

For experienced practitioners, making assessments along these dimensions is almost second nature. Less experienced practitioners who use this assessment approach may need to work harder to get a meaningful understanding of personality dynamics, especially regarding matters that are out of the patient's conscious awareness.

How Does the Person Manage Reality?

Reality testing is the oldest standard criterion used to differentiate psychotic from nonpsychotic states. Does the person know what is real and what is not real? Is the person delusional, hallucinating? Short of a frank psychosis, however, it is more common for a person to carry within the self an encapsulated pocket of reality distortion of greater or lesser magnitude, depending on the current circumstances. The significance of the misreading or misattribution of reality leaks (or bursts) out of the capsule and becomes evident when the person is under duress.

Judy (described at the beginning of the chapter) had a crisis when she did not know what was happening to her. She confused the difference between her fears and imaginings about her body and the indications of reality. At the time of her last hospitalization, she was so anxious about her well-being that she became convinced she was dying. On another occasion, Judy made an appointment for an office visit, thinking she had an ear infection. While the physician was examining her, a staff member notified him of an urgent telephone call from the hospital. He excused himself and left the room for 5 minutes. When he returned, Judy was in tears. She thought he left the room because what he saw in her ear was so bad that he did not want to tell her about it. Her ideas of reference confused her repeatedly, and she had difficulty believing that external events were not necessarily related to her. Judy sees the world through and around pockets of distortion. When she was particularly anxious, her fantasies filled up so much of her internal space that she was unable to relate to the world outside of herself. It was not always possible to predict when the line between anxiety-driven fantasy and florid delusion would be crossed.

Judy had a schizotypal personality disorder. She was globally eccentric, socially uncomfortable, and subject to cognitive and perceptual alterations that distort consensual reality. For most of her life, she had been able to establish the necessary barriers and compromises between her internal reality and the reality requirements of the outside world. She even used diabetes as a distancing device, to withdraw from others when the need arose, to "rest." When pressed hard by family problems, however, her regulatory capacities failed her and she became overwhelmed. During those periods, she lost her grip on reality (eccentric at the best of times), and her magical beliefs about health and illness took on a delusional quality.

How Does the Person Manage Anxiety?

Anxiety is a given in human experience, from a mild flutter to overwhelming dread of annihilation. The assault of disease on the body stimulates anxiety. The internal management of anxiety requires multiple processes to assess and handle both mild and extraordinary threat from within and without the person. Perhaps the most important dimension to consider under this question is the capacity to bear feelings—to regulate the affect, impulses, and drives as they ebb and flow. How comfortable is the person with anger, dependency, conflict, ambiguity, change? At what point does the presence of strong feeling, in and of itself, provoke anxiety?

Defenses protect people from anxiety. Therefore, the practitioner wants to know which defenses an individual uses. How adaptive are the defenses? How brittle? How primitive? If higher order defenses fail, what defenses remain for the person to draw on? What combinations and evolutions of defense patterns are available for anxiety reduction?

The threshold of a stimulus barrier provides another marker for the understanding of anxiety management. How quickly is the person overwhelmed by stress? What are the particular tolerances for excitation or deprivation? The stimulus barrier is related to the defensive operations, but it is also a function of inborn temperament (and probably the imprint of heritable physiology, too). Culture and developmental stage may strongly influence the threshold for tolerance of various stimuli. Stimulus threshold can be a vital variable for people with chronic illnesses, that is, how strongly a person perceives or manages pain.

All four of the diabetic patients presented had struggles with high levels of anxiety. Denise had a preexisting characterologically defensive eating habit. When threatened by interpersonal conflict or loss of a relationship, she fed herself. Such an important defense was itself threatened by the intrusion of diabetic dietary requirements. The conflict between her need to eat and her need not to eat (in the impulse-ridden habitual way) was not resolvable, so she blotted out the reality with denial. Her anxiety was increased greatly by her family members' progressive disability and death from the same disease. As a result, she increased the denial to global proportions.

Prior to the onset of diabetes, Denise already functioned with a borderline personality organization. She had marked instability of mood, relationships, and self-image. She had little ability to regulate her feelings and impulsivity, particularly when anxiety about separation and abandonment was stirred. When distressed by an argument with a sister or lover, Denise threw caution to the wind and ate until she felt better. Before psychotherapy, she had no other reliable way to diminish or tolerate negative feelings. Diabetes, with its devastating impact on her and her family, intensified her anxiety from the separation level to the annihilation level. Serious illness can push any person to the deepest levels of anxiety. The more fragile the personality structure, the more likely the person will fragment with the intensifying levels of anxiety.

Richard's premorbid level of adaptation was much higher than Denise's or Judy's functioning. He had more resources with which to handle anxiety, organized around an obsessive–compulsive personality. He was an orderly perfectionist who had a relatively secure sense that his life was under control until the onset of diabetes. On diagnosis, it did not seem surprising that he would take charge of the situation, making good use of his intellect and self-discipline to manage the illness. Over time, however, the conflict between his need for control and the reality that he could not control diabetes (although he could control his diet and exercise and thereby have an influence on the course of the disease) raised his anxiety to the point where he was suffering from a full-blown obsessive–compulsive disorder. Richard's predominant defenses against anxiety were the undoing and the isolation of affect. He did not process feelings directly and consciously, nor did he discuss his feelings or fears with anyone. He was unaware of the connection between his escalating obsessive and compulsive symptoms and his warding off of feelings. With no way to work through his dilemma and to accept his feelings and impulses (except to redouble his efforts at control), his defenses began to fail him. His emergency room visits were expressions of stimulus barrier breech and defense breakdown: The attempts at magically undoing the disease did not work any longer; the intrusive thoughts of impending serious illness took over, and his anxiety could not be contained with his customary resources. Unfortunately, instead of turning to his fiancée for emotional support, he drove her away in the attempt to rid himself of emotionality and vulnerability. It was not until he entered psychotherapy and reconnected his own emotionality to its rightful place in his life that he was able to reconnect with her.

Marion initially seemed to resemble Richard in her personality style. In fact, her record keeping of blood sugars was more thorough at the outset. It took some time for a truer picture of her depressive personality structure to emerge. When her anxiety mounted and her defenses gave way, she revealed the depressive core that had been hidden by the many rituals, charts, and graphs.

How Does the Person Manage Relationships?

The question about relationship management relates to conscious present relationships and to unconscious internal object relations based on early relational experiences. It encompasses the assessment of a person's capacity for age-appropriate, give-and-take relationships. Illness may alter participation, dependence–independence levels, and role function with other people, which can be burdensome to the patient or the other person. Therefore, practitioners must inquire about the nature and quality of the patient's object relations before illness, if possible. Are they mature or characterized by primitive, undifferentiated, infantile, merged relating? For example, a mature person with significant disability and necessary dependence on a caretaker may nevertheless be able to acknowledge readily the caretaker's need for time away from caregiving duties. In that case, there is room for the needs of both parties. The person who operates at an undifferentiated level of object relations, regardless of the presence or absence of illness, cannot perceive the needs of the other as distinct from his or her own needs. Of course, many people fall elsewhere on the primitive–mature continuum.

Other dimensions for assessment are intensity, duration, and constancy of object relations. Many a psychotherapist has been unpleasantly surprised by the difference between what a patient knows consciously about his or her relational world and the intense intrapsychic object world enacted in the transference–countertransference relationship that takes place in the consulting room.

Marion's primary relationship was with a husband who was emotionally and physically abusive to her. Her ability to set limits with him over the course of the marriage had improved somewhat, but his attitude toward her remained critical and undermining. Why would she sustain this kind of relationship?

The answer lies in its striking resemblance to her parents' marriage and her childhood relationship with her father, a critical and punishing man who told her directly and repeatedly that she was bad (for wanting, doing, being) and who took a similar tone with his wife. Her mother was a woman with low self-esteem, who died of the complications of diabetes. Because her mother did not protect her from her father's angry demanding personality style, Marion assumed for a long time that her mother shared his opinion of her. The mother seems to have expected Marion (and herself) to placate the father and give up hope for the normal, expectable quotient of parental support that is necessary for adequate emotional development. The mother, in all likelihood, had a depressive personality, too, which Marion had incorporated and, through identification, had made her own.

When Marion was wringing her hands and confessing her badness to the physician for not following the diabetic diet and exercise program, she was giving voice to the harsh punitive introject of her father. Additionally, the old object relation was overlaid with the power of a daily reinforcer in the person of her husband. Turning against herself (a frequently used depressive defense) enabled her to hold on to her significant relationships internally. In that way, she could attack the waves of vulnerability and helplessness stimulated by the disease and try to ignore her wishes for encouragement and reassurance and her anger at having to bear a burden that seemed too heavy.

Denise's relationships were colored by her use of splitting as a defense. In her object relations world, people were either all good or all bad. There were occasional intense and sudden shifts, when she was offended, and a formerly good object became a bad one. Denise viewed her parents as perfectly good, without fault. She told her physician she would do anything in her power for them. She viewed her sisters as bad, lazy, and uncaring about her parents. The men Denise dated were idealized as wonderful or skewered as wretched. The splitting defense was evident with physicians, too; those who fell from her good graces were on her rejection list, never to be seen again.

It is interesting to note that on occasion Denise was able to form a perception of her daughter as "all right," which showed a more neutral assessment that could contain both good and bad elements. This phenomenon reflected her limited differentiation from her daughter and expressed a statement about herself as well as the relationship to her offspring. During her psychotherapy, the starting position for the development of an enhanced self that could tolerate negative affects was that set of fleeting experiences in holding good and bad together, without flying apart psychically.

Judy's relationships were characterized by distance. Her primary complaint was that her husband wanted her to join him in activities and spend more time with him. Overall, she had trained her family quite well in regard to her need for interpersonal distance. Her 30-year history of diabetes was particularly useful, because she had conveyed to the family her frequent need to withdraw and rest to prevent making the diabetes worse. The family respected her wishes. Just prior to the hospitalization when Judy decompensated and lost her hold on reality, her extended family and friends gathered at her house for a reunion. She was very anxious about possible close contact and social demands during that period and was unable to find a way to withdraw into her own world and escape from people.

Richard related through, around, by, and with control. He had high standards for himself and for others. His need for control was so great that he sacrificed a primary relationship in his quest to regain the control that was slipping away from him. Because he actively avoided discussions of relationships and feelings, less is known about his early object history than those of the other three diabetic patients. The physician was not privy to this realm, and the psychologist was bound by Richard's need to keep the narrative of his early history somewhat sparse and matter of fact.

How Does the Person Manage Cognition?

Cognition management encompasses thought processing style (breadth, clarity, attention span, effectiveness); judgment capacities (consideration of consequences); autonomous mental functions (perceptual, motor, verbal); and synthetic–integrative functions (the ability to see the forest and not just the trees). Disturbances in any of these areas can interfere with adaptive response to illness. There is, however, a wide range of cognitive styles, and no one mode of cognitive operation need take precedence.

When people are given bad news, they respond at their own pace and level of assimilation. For example, when told that they require heart bypass surgery, a mastectomy, or permanent use of a wheelchair, some people cry out, some fall numb and silent, some ask a lot of questions immediately, and some go away and return later with their questions. There are patients whose anxiety is reduced and controlled by seeking and obtaining medical information. There are others whose anxiety is heightened by the availability of too much medical information for them to process comfortably. Each patient has to titrate his or her own dosage of information about the disease or condition, although psychological practitioners can be of assistance in helping patients and physicians arrive at a manageable balance.

Both Denise and Judy had cognitive problems. Denise, a concrete and compartmentalized thinker, did not synthesize and integrate concepts into a whole. She was unable to generalize learning: When she eventually understood that it was important to substitute roasted fish or poultry for fried, she could not generalize the principle to potatoes. In her mind, vegetables were in a different category from meats, and so the addition of fats and oils did not enter into her thinking. Once the psychologist had identified the cognitive problem, the physician and dietitian were able to devise a highly specific and detailed list of food choices, eating schedules, and insulin schedules, which Denise could actually follow.

Judy's thought processes were filled with loose associations, magical correlations, and irrational assumptions. She spent hours attempting to identify exactly which stressor or combination of stressors caused her blood sugar to vary (something many individuals with diabetes try to ascertain on a more rational scale). In the middle of the night Judy would ruminate about the causes of an elevation: perhaps it was related to a dream that woke her, or maybe the fruit salad she ate the night before, or maybe insufficient exercise the previous day, or maybe an item that was worrying her about the next day. Depending on which idea was dominant at the time, she would reduce or increase the physician's recommended dose of insulin, hoping to get the right blood sugar level. All of this information was recorded carefully, with some entries coded in blue ink, some in black, red, green, and so forth. One physician struggled to make sense of her system for years, without recognizing the underlying bizarre nature of her thinking.

Richard was a clear thinker with good judgment normally. In fact, his many strong cognitive capacities contributed to his success as a scientist. He was quite capable of using intellectualism as a defense against the messy domain of affect. Under the strain of illness he became increasingly anxious, divorced from his feelings and impulses, and withdrawn from sources of social support. When he could not stop the intrusive and interfering thoughts, he started to feel assaulted and betrayed by his own mind. His judgment about the validity of his exaggerated fears about infections and colds during this period was poor.

What Is the Person's Mastery–Competence Level?

The question about a person's mastery–competence level summarizes the overall picture of personality and the effects of illness. Small (1979) has explained this dimension as "the relationship between the individual's capacity and his actual mastery of his environment, the degree of congruence between feelings of competence and manifest competence" (p. 96).

The *Diagnostic and Statistical Manual of Mental Disorders* (4th ed., American Psychiatric Association, 1994), commonly called the *DSM–IV*, provides a widely used Global Assessment of Functioning (GAF) Scale (p. 32). The GAF scale is a continuum from 0 to 100 that encompasses psychological, social, and occupational functioning, to be used with any patient, regardless of disorder. It is not specific to patients with physiologically based diseases and conditions, but it has its roots in Luborsky's (1962) Health–Sickness Rating Scale. Many practitioners (and third-party payer gatekeepers) rely on the GAF continuum to convey a total impression.

If there are disjunctures between a patient's psychological capacity to function and his or her actual performance, practitioners must understand the source of the interference. Is the interference a function of the disease or a function of the personality? In many instances, the answer lies in the interaction between the two. For example, Marion's depressive personality style led her repeatedly back to sad, berating attacks on herself. On the other hand, the demand characteristics of diabetes are very strong. No one can follow a strict regimen of regulating food and exercise day in and day out, without feeling constrained, rebellious, discouraged, worried about advancement of the disease, and jealous of nonpatients (for their freedom) and of other diabetic patients (for their better control). Perfect mastery, perfect compliance without interruption, is not possible. Marion needed a more positive loving introject to counter the critical introject. She was capable of managing her disease adequately but needed support during her periods of natural discouragement and psychic fatigue with the onerous process of disease management. Without support, she relapsed into childlike collapsed states.

Is the interference of disease likely to be permanent or time-limited until the patient can adjust and reassemble a new pattern of function? Many patients experience an acute crisis stage when diagnosed with a serious disease and suffer a temporary decrement in function. For example, the early weeks after a diagnosis of cancer are a time of turmoil, and it is a mistake to assume that exaggerated personality responses are predictive of eventual ability to cope and reorganize. Other time-limited responses may last longer and appear less acute, such as the period of depression that often occurs when a person learns he or she will never walk, or hear, or see again.

Summary

The individual character styles of four diabetic patients have been presented to illustrate the personality structure themes. Assessment features include personality type, functional capacities, trait factors, ego functions, and personal hierarchies. The Psychological Template is presented as the frame for personality structure and functioning and is the fourth template in the holographic view of illness.

Practitioners use their assessment of patients' discrete and aggregate physical, psychological, and social competencies to inform their treatment plans. Both patients and psychotherapists want the treatments to work, but there is wide variance in the tolerance for slow progress, for setbacks, for trial and error. How can we improve the chances for a successful outcome? Good psychotherapy requires an understanding of the illness, the patient's response to the illness, and the patient's personality functions and individual history.

II

Treating Chronic Illness

5

Psychological Treatment Strategies

By the time a person perceives that an illness is chronic, the threats and assaults to the body and mind have become familiar terrain. The daily management of these assaults and indignities takes on the coloration of the familiar, often long before the psychological implications and consequences are understood. In the preceding chapters we have been constructing a hologram of the patient with chronic illness: with multiple views of disease, of personality, and of the threat and response process. The multidimensional holographic "picture" provides the depth of information required to develop effective psychotherapeutic treatment approaches. We turn now to applications.

Overview of Treatment

The shared treatment tasks of the patient and the therapist are as follows: (a) facing the problem of intrapsychic disorganization (the challenge to self and identity); (b) working through the reorganization, the reshaping of a changed self (according to coping resources and the illness trajectory); (c) achieving the desired outcome for the patient (reconsolidation of reconfigured self, stability of self in unstable body); and (d) providing a follow-up structure and process (to support the "hold" of the therapeutic work).

The focus on these tasks helps the patient move from the disorganizing early phases of the Response Template continuum to the adaptive reconsolidation phase

The therapist must tailor interventions to the personality resources of the patient and the press of the illness. This is the key to the effectiveness and responsiveness of any therapeutic treatment plan. If either the Medical Template or the Psychological Template is ignored, the treatment will founder. For example, a newly diagnosed breast cancer patient sought the assistance of a reputable psychotherapist in the community. She was in crisis, overwhelmed by the necessity of choosing among medical treatment options in a short period of time. Unfortunately, the therapist was oblivious to the particular press of the illness at the time. The patient needed help with the steep learning curve involved in gathering and translating medical information, assimilating the perceived threat to her life, assembling a support network, and making the practical arrangements required to cover work and family obligations. Her anxiety would have been better contained and reduced with this kind of focus. The therapist, who accurately assessed the precrisis resources of the woman, pursued a focus on the meaning and importance of the woman's breast. The patient left the therapist and sought another who was better able to recognize her present needs. Later, when she had moved through several phases in her adjustment and treatment (both medical and psychological), she was ready naturally to explore the personal meanings associated with her breasts. At the time of original crisis, however, she perceived her illness as acute and had not yet arrived at the internal realization of chronic alteration. In other words, she was in an acute stress phase of illness, not a chronic stress phase.

Treatment Strategies

The following treatment strategies are practical and should be of use to most practitioners. Some may need translation or modification to suit particular treatment orientations.

Obtain Sufficient Medical Information

The therapist must understand the choices and experiences confronting the patient. One need not become a medical expert, but it is important to become a knowledgeable consumer of medical information, as it becomes relevant to a general psychotherapy practice. It is fine to ask patients medical questions up to a point. That point is reached when you have reason to believe the patient's information is incomplete or distorted. The point is reached, too, when your need for information is burdensome to the patient, who should not have to experience a drag on psychological treatment while trying to educate the therapist. Last year, one of us (Carol Goodheart) received a call from a colleague requesting a therapist in a midwestern state with knowledge of childhood cancers. The family of the child consulted two psychotherapists with insufficient understanding of cancer and the sequelae of medical treatment, and they expressed an urgent need for a therapist who could fathom the child's experiences and the family's situation. Sometimes a specialist is called for, but in many instances, competent general practitioners can get sufficient supporting information.

1. Where can I find information? Start with chapter 2, which presents a schema for how to think about disease. It offers two templates for asking questions and organizing your understanding of illness and the important implications for your patients. In fact, if you photocopy the form and fill in the responses that you are able to obtain from the patient directly, you can then ask the patient's physician to fill in the missing pieces, in a time-efficient phone contact or facsimile exchange. The results will give you a baseline of necessary medical information, and the process can establish the beginning of treatment collaboration between physician and therapist. Chapter 11 provides a resource compilation of information on many specific diseases, from which you will be able to locate other resources as necessity and interest warrant.

2. When should I seek information? Obtain information whenever you have reason to believe a patient's disease is affecting his or her psychological functioning. For example, a young adult gay man came to psychotherapy complaining of relationship problems. He exhibited many risky behaviors in his flight from

anxiety states and his sexual patterns of relating, which were initially nonresponsive to treatment. One day he revealed a history of epilepsy, along with the information that he was not taking his anticonvulsant medication. The therapist did some pertinent reading on epilepsy before the next session. Then he was able to help the patient focus on the true source of the anxiety that had been driving the denial of his disease, the risky behavior, and the poor relational patterns. The patient was fleeing loss of control, shame, and rejection because of his epilepsy. The patient knew, and the therapist learned, of the stigma that epilepsy has carried for centuries (and still carries in some segments of society).

3. How should I seek information? Use "high tech" or old-fashioned methods to get the information you seek. It is helpful to the busy practitioner to gain information quickly, so you may find computer Internet resources a boon if you have access to them. Some automated information is available very quickly by facsimile transmission (e.g., see the description of CancerFax under the heading NCI—Cancer Information Service, in chapter 11), and some organizations fax summary information also. Medical reference librarians, who are highly skilled in technologically sophisticated methods of information transfer, are still the best resource for novice and experienced researchers alike. The government and many voluntary organizations such as the American Cancer Society, American Heart Association, and the National Arthritis Foundation all provide books, pamphlets, and other forms of information. Over time, you may build relevant medical information into your own library or file cabinet. For example, the first patient you treat who has multiple sclerosis may prompt a call to the National Multiple Sclerosis Society. The Society will send general or specific materials (e.g., on fatigue, pain, sexual dysfunction, medications), depending on the need. Thereafter, you have a ready reference in the office, although it must be updated from time to time.

Assess Response to Illness and Psychological Status

The patient's capacity to cope with and adapt to the disorganization caused by chronic illness will vary according to personality organization, life stage, maturational development, and internal resources (such as temperament and intelligence). The capacity to cope is tested also by the severity of the illness, its threat to life, and the extent of the disability. Anyone may develop a chronic illness. The range extends from normal people in abnormal circumstances to abnormal people in abnormal circumstances. An evaluation of the patient should include:

- identification of the type of illness (see chapter 2);
- location of the patient on a response continuum to the illness (see chapter 3);
- understanding of the patient's premorbid character structure (see chapter 4);
- knowledge of the patient's life stage, roles, and tasks (see chapter 7);
- availability of outside resources (family, money, community; see chapter 9).

It is essential for the therapist to grasp the problem of the disorganization process, of the narcissistic injury sustained, of the futile attempts to hold on to or return to the pre-illness self. Without that deeper understanding, the psychotherapist can see only the patient's surface of physical and emotional symptoms. For example, an intelligent and perceptive 57-year-old man was referred to a psychologist for noncompliance with simple home treatments (i.e., drinking sufficient water and taking a daily pill) for a relatively mild form of kidney disease. No amount of encouragement, exhortation, or exasperation on the part of the physician or wife produced the desired effect. The patient himself said he was puzzled about why he could not seem to take his condition seriously. Working together, the psychologist and patient arrived at a dynamic understanding of the patient's resistance: Acknowledgment of the presence of a chronic disease was being denied in order to avoid an anxiety constellation around aging, the possibility of becoming a burden to his family, and ultimately because of a deep-seated exaggerated fear of needing the help of others but of having that need resented and ignored by significant others. His underlying fear stemmed from his experience of unmet dependency needs in childhood, which had been successfully masked and compensated for during most of his masterful adult years. After the core anxiety was identified, the man was able to change his irrational response to the illness, although he elected to continue in psychotherapy to face concomitant anxieties about the impact of his aging process.

Integrate Theoretical Orientation and Illness

The therapist's theoretical orientation may be woven into a focus on the central shared tasks of treatment. Within the framework of addressing the continuum of disorganization, reorganization, and reconsolidation, it is possible for many styles of psychotherapy to coalesce. The psychodynamic–psychoanalytic therapist may add behavioral and educational components to the standard repertoire, and the cognitive–behavioral therapist may add self and object components to the standard repertoire. Similar cross-fertilization can occur with family systems therapists, feminist theory therapists, and others. In fact, it is likely that most therapists borrow from others anyway and offer an ever wider array of interventions as they grow and try to find approaches that benefit their patients.

Regardless of theoretical orientation, it can be clarifying and organizing for the therapist (thus, ultimately beneficial for the patient) to approach a conceptual understanding of the patient through the questions posed in chapter 4: How does the patient manage reality, anxiety, object relations, and cognitive functions, and what is the patient's mastery–competence level? This framework can be enlarged to encompass the therapist's customary ways of thinking about psychological functioning.

Offer a Menu of Interventions

The strategies above are to be used across the board. However, the selection of the following particular interventions is based on the changing needs and capacities of the patient and the experience and skill of the therapist. It is not possible within the limits of a chapter to explain in detail how to implement all the interventions referred to here. For example, most clinicians are trained to offer crisis management, but most are not trained to offer hypnosis for pain management. For further training in specific modalities, clinicians may turn to continuing education–training programs, such as that of the American Society for Clinical Hypnosis, which offers hypnosis training throughout the United States. All of the approaches have proved to be helpful, although one does not use all of them with any one patient. Conversely, no single approach is sufficient if used exclusively, except in rare circumstances.

1. Focused psychodynamic psychotherapy. This approach is based on empathic clarification, confrontation, and interpretation, as applied to feelings, defenses against feelings, and anxiety, in conjunction with past, present, and transference relationships. The reality and the personal meaning of the illness are explored; the internal disorganization is given voice; and the reorganization is worked through and lived through, until the goal of reconsolidation and a functional level of adaptation is achieved. Support for the grief reactions and mourning processes that accompany loss is an integral part of the approach. Support for frank discussion of body image, functioning, processes, and responses is also an integral part of the approach. Horowitz (1992) emphasized the central importance of using conscious awareness for change in doing brief psychotherapy for stress response syndromes. The consciousness is "used as a tool for unlearning automatic associations and resolving seemingly irreconcilable conflicts" (p. 99).

2. Crisis management. When the patient is flooded with affect and overwhelmed with anxiety and his or her ability to cope is compromised, the therapist selects crisis-oriented techniques. These revolve around the mobilization of internal and external resources for support and the shoring up of the defenses, until the patient can regain a sense of control.

3. Anxiety, pain, and cumulative stress reduction. These three areas overlap, and the presence of any one of them can trigger the appearance of another. Techniques to ameliorate one of them are often used with the others as well. This category includes psychoeducational techniques, cognitive–behavioral techniques, and emotive imaginative techniques. Examples are hypnosis, progressive relaxation, visualization, guided imagery, focused breathing, centering, assertiveness, and communication skills training. Specific to pain management is the use of pain scales, by which the patient rates the severity of the

pain and takes planned action to alleviate it depending on the severity.

4. Anger management. This approach, an adaptation of anxiety management training, uses guided imagery, anger arousal, and relaxation for self-control as methods to treat anger (Deffenbacher, Demm, & Brandon, 1986; Suinn, 1990, 1996). Dynamically oriented psychotherapists also may draw on their interpretive and "working through" skills to work with various styles of anger. For example, some men who have been reared to behave stoically are ashamed to reveal fears, so their primary defense against shame is anger. They simultaneously mask and express the anxiety with hostile aggressive behavior. Many therapists mix and match elements of dynamic, behavioral, and systems approaches according to the cause of the anger and functional style of the individual patient and the family.

We treated an out-of-control, angry, 37-year-old man with chronic lymphocytic leukemia. He was seen alone, in couples therapy with his wife, and in a coordinated treatment involving his children through their school-based community mental health program. The professionals involved included a psychologist, a physician, and a social worker, who drew on dynamic, behavioral, and systems interventions to defuse the explosive situation and improve coping ability. Specific interventions included the administration of antidepressant medication; the imagery–arousal–relaxation module mentioned in the previous paragraph; establishment of chore hierarchy for family members; a referral to a couples support group; and the provision of a mirroring, holding environment to contain his fragility. He was given a selection of audio tapes on visualization for cancer, encouraged to develop a pleasurable "safe place," and trained to use imagery and progressive relaxation.

5. Nonverbal psychotherapy techniques. Art therapy, sand play, and movement therapy are all examples of potentially therapeutic, nonverbal expressive treatment modalities. Such techniques can provide an alternative path to self-knowledge (for the patient) and another entry to understanding the experiential subjective world of the patient (for the psychotherapist). They are rarely used alone, but are more commonly added to other standard treatments. The visual, tactile, motile techniques are particu-

larly helpful with patients who have been traumatized; with patients who have learning disabilities; with patients who are stuck in a regressed, blocked, dissociated, or concrete state of functioning; and with children. Because body changes and body image changes are interior events, involving physical cues and perceptual cues, they often give rise to affects that are not readily accessible to verbal channels of information processing. It is more difficult for some patients than others to find the words to organize their experiences. (See chapter 7 for the clinical example of Gary, an asthmatic man with a fear of choking, whose symptoms responded dramatically to the experience of sand play.) Although some of the techniques are not easily used by practitioners without special training, equipment, or space, most psychotherapists can provide basic art materials, such as drawing paper and colored pencils, as an adjunct to psychological treatment.

6. Support for the patient's management of the illness. Many adjunctive regimens and alternative approaches to healing and to living better with illness are available. Therapists can support and encourage patients' efforts to contribute to their own well-being, without imposing judgment or personal values on their efficacy, unless they seem to be endangering themselves. Examples of such pursuits are personal illness diaries, exercise and nutrition programs, religious and spiritual participation, humorous tapes and books, and the alternative medicine movement.

7. Referral to support groups and community services. Patients who need professionally led psychotherapy groups are not candidates for this intervention. However, in addition to or after psychotherapy, many patients benefit from the companionship, shared experience, tips, and coping suggestions that may be found in support groups run by the American Cancer Society and other organizations. Community services such as transportation, housekeeping, equipment provision, and nursing assistance may ease the daily burden of patients.

8. Handling uncertainty and fear of death. Anxiety about the future is aroused by the intrusion of illness, a change in symptoms, a progression of the disease, a worsening of disability. Anxious fantasies can be aroused even when the patient does not feel sick or disabled but is "waiting for the time bomb to go off" (e.g., the dread of medical checkups for fear of bad news). Some

diagnoses—AIDS, cancer, heart disease—are particularly frightening. Harpham (1994) offered a practical framework for cancer survivors who struggle with cyclical checkup anxiety, which could be useful in other disease circumstances also. Her approach is based on framing the checkup as an opportunity to confirm that one is doing well and reinforcing the experience of a positive checkup.

Overall, the therapist must be sensitive to the patient's losses and fears about further loss, up to and including death. The therapist must provide a safety zone in the relationship, within which the patient is invited to discuss his or her uncertainty, wishes, and fears about dying. For the patient who needs another expressive pathway (in addition to the verbal one), the use of drawing, sand play, puppets, or toy figures provides an emotionally satisfying and therapeutic avenue (see No. 5 above)

The primary technique for death anxiety is to listen fully, which may be the most difficult technique of all to put into practice. To listen fully means to listen without judgment, without withdrawal, without denial, and without interference with the patient's hopes. To listen fully is to be present, with the patient, so that he or she is not alone in facing death.

Match the Psychological Focus of Intervention to the Need

In the overview section at the beginning of the chapter, the central focus of treatment was presented as the shared treatment tasks of the patient and the psychotherapist. Associated with the continuum of disorganization, reorganization, and reconsolidation, there are recurring themes in the emotional lives of patients, which often require a specific focus for psychological intervention. These themes lie between the layers of the continuum focus and the long list of possible symptoms that ebb and flow in individuals. The specific themes we have identified across many patients include (a) decreased self-esteem associated with body image changes; (b) mourning associated with loss; and (c) negative affects associated with physical, psychological, and social discomfort.

Treatment can be improved if clinicians look beyond the individual symptoms and help the patient link and resolve sub-symptoms with their larger themes. For example, both patient and clinician can become overwhelmed by a set of agitated depressive symptoms such as withdrawal, self-hatred, guilt, giving up, anger, and exacting from others. If a larger theme is identified (e.g., the stigma response constellation that is associated with facial disfiguration), then the focus of interpretation, strategy, and coping approaches is appropriately placed on the larger theme. After the larger salient focus has been identified, the reactive symptoms can be linked and addressed in the improved context. It is much more organizing, specific, and helpful to frame the poor self-esteem, grief, and anger within the context of stigma rather than to proceed merely with generic strategies for reactive depression.

Patients express their theme issues around self-esteem, mourning, and negative feelings in direct and indirect ways. Practitioners must be prepared to hear and focus on the following questions:

1. Will I be desirable? The arena may be sexual, social, or vocational, but the arena does not matter so much as the level of worry and reality. People who have been disfigured by surgery are often afraid they will not be attractive enough to find or hold an intimate sexual partner. People with disability are often afraid they will not be able to find or hold a satisfying job. Everyone must face rejection in life, but people with chronic diseases and conditions often face outright discrimination. Patients need an opportunity to sort through unfounded fears, blatant realities, and alternative paths to find acceptance in themselves and others.

2. Will I be able to . . .? Fill in the blank with the items that most people take for granted, but which chronically ill or disabled people cannot assume will be possible. Examples are: Will I be able to walk, return to school or work, have sex, adjust to a wheelchair or a limited diet or the total absence of sound? Will I have the stamina to get through an ordinary day?

3. Will I be free of . . .? People want to know if improvement is possible. They are often fearful about how they will manage if their condition worsens. Common concerns are: Will I be free of pain, flare-ups, limitations in movement or stamina, anxiety about my body?

4. How can I live like this? Patients with limited coping resources before the onset of illness are apt to become overwhelmed and overtaxed by their condition early on in the disease process. Even people who cope quite well have their discouraged, tired moments or periods. At those times, patients ask us how can they possibly live with reduced financial circumstances, disability, pain, terror about recurrences or progression of disease, or with the knowledge that there is no known cure.

Sensitive practitioners can be prepared for these kinds of questions. Sometimes one follows patients (when they take the lead in grappling with acknowledged questions), and sometimes one leads the patients (when they need help to identify or articulate the pressing themes). Most of the time, practitioners pace the patients (when they need a partner, ally, and calm presence to work through these difficult questions, problems, and challenges).

Face the Countertransference Responses

Just as patients have transferences and their illnesses have personal meanings, so do therapists have countertransferences and their patients' illnesses stir personal meanings. Perhaps the most common therapist reaction to treating a chronically ill patient is anxiety, which in a high-functioning therapist is managed through a goodly number of defenses. Countertransference difficulties tend to be greatest with a dying patient, although this is not universally true.

Therapists should ask themselves: Do I have any feelings about this patient (or myself when I am with this patient) that interfere with my ability to be neutral? A neutral stance does not mean an uncaring or uninvolved attitude; it means that the therapist should not have an agenda for the patient. That is, the patient must not be required to get well, be brave, be a fighter, stop complaining, change personality traits—in short, to change anything in order to meet the therapist's needs. Definitions, typical inductions, examples, and problems of countertransference are discussed in greater depth in chapter 6.

Treatment Focus Examples

Four diabetic patients (Denise, Richard, Marion, and Judy) with differing personality organizations were introduced in the previous chapter. Here their treatment is highlighted, in order to illustrate the tailoring of interventions to personality resources and the press of the illness. The brief sketches omit much background; our intent is to illustrate the dynamic focus with illness for each of them rather than to offer full case explications.

Denise

Overview: Denise's mother and sister both died of complications of diabetes within 18 months of her psychotherapy treatment. Denise's own disease was progressive, her kidneys were failing, and her physician informed her that renal dialysis was mandatory to save her kidney function and preserve her life. She refused.

Personality organization: Borderline personality disorder with narcissistic features.

Defenses: Primitive, nonadaptive, breaking down. Omnipotence and denial present ("What happened to mother and sister can't happen to me," binge eating despite consequences to health, refusal to consider dialysis).

Functioning: Denise demonstrated high anxiety, poor impulse control, concrete cognitive style with inability to follow abstractions, and volatile object relations.

Treatment focus: The focal strategies were containment, addressing the cognitive deficit, and working through her mourning. When the therapist confronted Denise clearly and gently with her functioning, anxiety, and consequences, the interventions served to organize and contain her anxiety and (thus) her wild self-destructive actions. She "firmed up" and was relieved rather than wounded by the directness of the therapist. (It probably made a difference, too, that the particular therapist had a warm and gentle manner.) The cognitive deficit was noticeable in her poor synthetic–integrative function, impaired judgment, and concrete thinking. Therefore, psychotherapeutic clarifications and interpretations had to be concrete to match her learning disability in order for her to understand them. To release the grief and enable mourning for family losses, the therapist helped Denise to label what she was going through, offering empathy for her experiences and helping her to differentiate herself from her mother and sister. The therapist helped her to increase her tolerance for negative feelings long enough to do something other than to eat destructively. Concretely, Denise had feared the dialysis procedures would kill her, because her family members had both died after dialysis, although she had a much better medical prognosis. Collaboration between the physician and therapist was productive. The therapist gained valuable medical information about Denise's physical problems and needs. The physician had been quite frustrated with Denise's noncompliance with medical treatment recommendations. He learned to be more straightforward and concrete when he talked with her, to write down concrete instructions and facts, and to check on her understanding of them.

Outcome: In the end, Denise was able to mourn, separate, lessen her anxiety, and understand as much as was necessary for her to undergo renal dialysis and to improve her health and her life.

Richard

Overview: On the surface, and to his physician, Richard appeared to be handling his diabetes very well. By following a careful regimen, he had his blood sugars under meticulous control. He was well educated and held a high-level responsible job.

Personality organization: Obsessive–compulsive structure.

Defenses: The predominant protections Richard had been able to use successfully for most of his life were not holding anxiety at bay any longer. They were isolation of affect (the separation of thoughts from feelings) and undoing (the unconscious attempts to eradicate diabetes). He tried to protect himself with compulsive behavioral regimens.

Functioning: Intrusive obsessions drove Richard to seek psychotherapy. He was increasingly preoccupied with thoughts of illness; for example, he worried that a common cold might become pneumonia and that a small cut could develop into a serious infection. His compulsive behaviors that surrounded the regulation of blood sugars, diet, and exercise did not trouble him, but they were occupying more and more of his day.

Treatment focus: The central tenet of Richard's sense of self was rational control of himself and of his world. Diabetes is a disease that thwarts that sense of control; medical treatment regimens are predicated on attempts to bring the disease under control. That tension is difficult for anyone, but for Richard it was his greatest threat. The key dynamic psychotherapy strategies involved facing the loss of control and helping him to reintegrate his hidden affect. First, the fears about loss of control had to be clarified. Then he was able to raise his fears about disability and death. He gained more access to the feeling side of himself as he came to understand the relationship between his undoing and his walled-off emotions.

Outcome: The obsessions diminished markedly, the compulsive behaviors loosened somewhat, and he regained his sense of balance. After coming to grips with his fears, he was better able to live with the diabetes. He worked his way through to a reconsolidation of self, with the ability to tolerate somewhat less control and somewhat more emotionality.

Marion

Overview: Marion presented an uneven picture in handling her diabetes. She alternated between extremes. For periods of time, she would rigidly manage with compulsive charting of blood sugars, exercise, and diet. However, she was more brittle than Richard, and therefore she would collapse under stress. Her background contains abuse by both her father, now dead, and her husband, with whom she lives. Her mother died of the same disease.

Personality organization: Depressive core, with an obsessive–compulsive surface.

Defenses: Introjection (not initially visible to the therapist until she witnessed the collapsed Marion berating herself with the cruel tones of her father) was at the root. The more readily apparent compulsions and rigidities were attempts to pull herself together and take care of herself, assuming there were no other reliable caretakers available.

Functioning: Marion was a sad woman, for whom the diabetes was an overwhelming burden. Before the onset of diabetes, she had undergone long-term psychotherapy with significant improvement. The illness created a crisis for her, and she had regressed to her pretherapy level of functioning, in which she would cry, wring her hands, withdraw, and tell her physician, "I know it's [the diabetes] going to get me."

Treatment focus: The most important strategies were to address her unmet dependency needs and to support her right to proper care. As a child, she had nowhere to turn for consistent comfort and support. She came to the erroneous conclusion, as abused children so often do, that she was bad and undeserving (the cruel introjected parental message). The first therapy had not confronted her neediness at such a basic level. Therefore, in the present treatment, the therapist had to help her uncover and face her anxieties about being helpless and without hope of help from others. The task was easier to accomplish than under most circumstances, because Marion had a successful previous psychotherapy on which to draw. The work involved a reweaving, another reconsolidation for her, while this time taking into account her illness and her deep-seated depressive core. In addition, the therapist referred her to yoga classes. These added group support and enhanced her body image, enabling her to participate more consistently in the exercise program recommended for diabetic control.

Outcome: Marion improved considerably, gaining a belief that she is "entitled" to take good care of herself (managing her diabetic routines) and to ask others for their assistance and support, too. She remained vulnerable to losing that belief temporarily under duress but was able to regain her equilibrium with support. The therapist alerted the physician to Marion's need for consistency of support, and Marion was assigned a "support" staff person in the physician's office, who spent time with her during routine office visits. Behaviorally, Marion learned to set limits on her husband. She no longer tolerated verbal sniping and tongue lashings.

Judy

Overview: This elderly woman with long-standing diabetes was a puzzle to her physician. Judy would bring books of diabetic record keeping to the physician, but on close examination they seemed to bear no rhyme or reason. Judy was testing her blood sugars up to 10 times a day, unrelated to eating schedules, sometimes in the middle of the night. Judy's explanation was that stress causes blood sugars to vary, so she expected hers to vary. One day, Judy became incoherent in the physician's office and was hospitalized for a major physical workup (for heart disease, stroke, etc.). All findings were normal. Throughout this period all blood sugars were normal. During the hospital respite, Judy's confusion and disorganization lifted. After this episode the physician referred her to a psychologist for psychological evaluation.

Personality organization: Schizotypal personality disorder, with periodic decompensation into psychotic states when severely strained and overtaxed by emotional demands.

Defenses: Withdrawal into her own inner world and the establishment of a carefully regulated distance from others allowed Judy enough comfort to function under normal circumstances. She maintained her inner world with bizarre notions and constructions and with self-referential thinking as a way to process outside events when necessary.

Functioning: A loner, Judy managed to have a family and community life by maintaining the ties with a "very long cord that allows me to go around the corner and stay to myself." Most people, including her physician, were not aware of her magical thinking patterns and lapses into looseness of organization. When intruded on by family members' problems that became too upsetting to ignore, her distancing regulation would fail, and she would become overstimulated, overwhelmed, and anxious. In attempting to escape the intrusive threat, her internal fanciful world lost its connection to the external world, and she exhibited a florid thought disorder until safety could be restored. Judy's responses to her long-standing diabetes were a reflection of her overall psychological functioning. Her management of the disease was usually adequate but was susceptible to increasingly dysfunctional patterns as she lost her hold on reality.

Treatment focus: The therapist's goal was to help Judy regain and maintain her optimal level of functioning as established over a lifetime. Therefore, the primary focus was on the regulation and decrease of stressful experiences before they reached intolerable levels. The therapist interpreted, and Judy was able to understand, the cycle of overstimulation, overwhelmed response, regression into confusion, and disorganization. Building on that, they were able to implement useful strategies. Judy learned when and how to say no and to establish firmer boundaries in the real world (not just in her fantasy world). She learned to set limits on others' claims on her emotional resources and time. The therapist worked with the physician to provide additional psychological supports along with the medical maintenance. They included anti-anxiety medication for use during particularly stressful periods and direct reassurance during physician visits. For example, Judy once believed the physician was conveying the message that the diabetes was worsening, because the physician was late in returning a telephone call. In the subsequent visit, the physician had to reassure her that her diabetes had not worsened.

Outcome: Judy's functioning improved. Her disintegrative periods were fewer, less severe, and less long lasting. She returned to checking her blood sugars only three times a day (the norm).

Summary

This chapter presents an overview of psychological treatment that focuses on the shared tasks of treatment. Associated with the continuum of disorganization and reconsolidation are the themes of decreased self-esteem, mourning, and negative affects. Treatment strategies include obtaining sufficient medical information, assessing response to illness and psychological status, integrating theoretical orientation and illness, and offering a menu of interventions to fit the patient's needs. Four patients were used as case illustrations. Each of the four patients needed an individually tailored treatment based on their personality, disease threat, and response to diabetes. For Denise, psychotherapy was primarily cognitive management of her deficits and working through her grief processes. Richard's treatment was primarily dynamic and involved the reintegration of his repressed affect. Marion's treatment was a combination of dynamic insight, cognitive strategies, and fundamental support for her dependency needs. Judy's treatment was primarily the provision of a supportive structure and the regulation of her stressful experiences. Each patient experienced significant internal disorganization, but with psychotherapy, all of them showed improved adaptation to the demands of their disease and greater stability of self. Collaboration between the physician and the psychologist was helpful for the long-term support of the therapeutic gains, particularly for Denise and Judy.

Chapter 6

Countertransference

Psychotherapy with patients who have chronic debilitating illnesses seeds a particularly fertile field of countertransference "growth" in therapists. There are many varieties of seeds and qualities of soil. The reactive growth may be characterized by borrowing images from the plant world, such as small groundcovers, mixed perennial borders, waves of grain, stinky weeds, exotic hybrids, delicate flowers, sweeps of lawn, barren patches, common houseplants, formal parterres, insect-infested plants, fragrant herb gardens, and the like. The metaphoric diversity of the botanical habitats indicates the multiplicity of countertransference habitats to be understood and acknowledged.

An understanding of the concept of countertransference provides both an enhanced experience of the self for the therapist to cultivate and a useful tool in the therapeutic relationship. Awareness of countertransference, the broad strokes and nuances alike, gives information about the texts and subtexts of the psychotherapy that is not available in any other form. Thus, it is a fruitful way of thinking for all therapists to consider, whether or not a given therapist would describe himself or herself as working within a psychodynamic focus.

Definitions

Patients initiate, relate, and respond to the reality of the therapist's role and personality style, and they initiate, relate, and respond according to their lifelong, internal, fantasied expectations of the other person. In other words, most patients create a mixture of reality and transference in their reactions to their therapists. Occasionally, patients are unable to take in the reality components on a reliable or consistent basis, which complicates the treatment by making the therapeutic alliance precarious. Therapists, in turn, participate in a therapeutic relationship by conscious and unconscious design as well. They have countertransference reactions to the style and problems of their patients, which are shaped by their own history and personality, as well as any fantasied expectations that may be triggered by the patients' mode of relating or the patients' illnesses.

A classic definition of countertransference is "the whole of the analyst's unconscious reactions to the individual analysand—especially to the analysand's own transference" (LaPlanche & Pontalis, 1973, p. 92). Originally, countertransference manifestations were considered an impediment to treatment, a sign of leftover unanalyzed remnants of the analyst's life, to be eliminated if possible. It was expected that a patient would have a transference to the analyst, but the analyst's neutrality demanded a blank screen in return.

Today, dynamically oriented psychotherapists and theoreticians are likely to view countertransference phenomena in a more positive light. They view it as an aid to understanding the patient's experience through the therapist's own personality filter. The relational matrix of transference and countertransference responses is similar to "call and response" singing, in which the basic song is varied and sometimes even created anew by the influences of caller and responder on each other.

Perhaps a note of caution is in order here. Competent ethical therapists do not merely spill a spontaneous countertransference reaction into the treatment. They interpose an intermediary step by analyzing the reaction before translating the response into a form that patients can hear and use. For example, therapists do not blurt out feelings of boredom, despair, attraction, disgust, rescuing, and the like, because they are hurtful. In addition, they do not initially understand what has been created in the relational matrix and why. When the understanding has been achieved, an effective, on-target course of action in the treatment is possible.

Induced Responses

Two classes of induced countertransference are of significant relevance to chronically ill patients: (a) responses to the disease impact and its usual course and (b) responses to the individual patient's characterological reactions to the disease.

Patients with non–life-threatening waxing and waning illnesses of unknown etiology (such as chronic fatigue syndrome) are most likely to induce a sense of uncertainty about the nature of the illness. Therapists may find themselves questioning the reality of the illness, the severity of the symptoms, the source of the dysfunction. Is she sick or not sick? Is he crazy or sick? Is this psychosomatic in origin? This process parallels the patient's search for certainty. It is a natural response to an ambiguous set of psychophysiological conditions.

Patients with known progressive life-threatening illnesses are most likely to induce responses to the magnitude of the losses and fears. Therapists vary in their capacity to work with a dying patient, just as patients vary in their ability to face death. The parallel process in this instance includes the struggle between hope and despair, helplessness and control, anxiety and comfort, depression and transcendence.

In response to patients' particular characterological reactions to their illnesses, therapists often know they are susceptible to liking the "good" patient and disliking or trying to escape from the "bad" patient. It is easy to admire the patient who shows spunk, tries hard to make use of help, never shows anger at being sick, but is appropriately angry and assertive with "other" caregivers. Conversely, it is easy to feel hateful toward patients who cannot contain their affective responses to the disease process but dump all of their fury, sadism, contempt, and manipulations into their therapists' laps.

Comparison: One Patient and Three Therapists' Countertransferences

A 45-year-old woman, Mary, is referred to a male therapist. She has recently completed treatment for breast cancer, which included a lumpectomy, radiation therapy, and chemotherapy. With a hopeful posttreatment prognosis, she had expected to feel relieved and to "get on" with her life, resuming her old familiar patterns of life. Instead, she finds herself with uncomfortable symptoms: fatigue, anxiety, intrusive thoughts about her treatment experiences, self-absorption, conflict with her partner, quick to cry and get angry over minor frustrations. She is upset and surprised with herself for feeling depressed. She knew she would feel intermittent dread about a recurrence but had not expected all the rest of her symptoms.

On the surface, the male therapist responds with seeming interest, competence, and humanity, all of which are true components of his personality. Now imagine three different therapists and their guiding internal experiences.

One of the therapists, John, lost his mother to breast cancer when she was 47 years old, after treatment, remission, relapse, and further treatment did not halt the disease progression. John is apt to be pulled into a maternal transference to Mary; that is, he experiences her and relates to her as though she were his mother, even though he knows rationally that she is not his mother and is expected to have a different outcome. His countertransference is shaped by his awareness of his internal fantasy; his personal style of defensive organization, object relations, and ego strength; and on the quality of the relationship he had with his mother. He may have mourned his mother's death and worked through the loss of his parent, or the grief may be in progress, or it may be unresolved. He may live out a reparative healing fantasy with his patient, a revenge fantasy, a rescuing fantasy. He may deny, split, dissociate, minimize, exaggerate, fuse, acknowledge, or grapple with the coincidence of the two women. Yet, no matter where he falls on the continuum of response, his history will be a part of the present therapy. It will be in the fabric of the therapeutic relationship, although he will never tell Mary anything about his own life experiences.

Another therapist, Martin, is a conscientious and able man who is somewhat obsessive–compulsive in his style of organization. Faced with anxiety-provoking situations, he would not ordinarily succumb to helplessness or even experience helplessness consciously. Instead, he tends to use his ideas and intellect to mobilize attempts to solve anxiety-inducing problems. In the main, this is adaptive for him, and he is known to be quite creative in developing strategic ideas for coping. He brings his considerable energies to the treatment of Mary and is most likely to be helpful to her in devising ways for her to move forward. A potential countertransference problem will arise, however, if he cannot truly hear, absorb, and contain her strongest affective experiences, because her feelings represent the primary problem that is driving her to seek psychological help. If he cannot fathom her fears and his own, and face helplessness, he will be increasingly cut off from the related affective world of loss, grief, pain, anxiety, and trauma. If that occurs, the treatment will fail. He may join her in her presenting expectation to "get on" with life without mastering the experiential impact and personal meaning of the illness. He may disengage from her to avoid a subjective experience of helplessness. He may devalue her as a weak woman ruled by feelings instead of reason. He may redouble his own efforts and exhort her to try harder to implement coping strategies. All of these responses are typical countertransference problems elicited by the circumstances of a dissonance between the patient's needs and the therapist's needs.

A third therapist, Robert, is in the midst of a divorce process at the time of the referral. He is very aware of the toll his personal crisis has been taking on him and, therefore, makes every effort to put it aside while he is working. Nevertheless, he is vulnerable to a countertransference storm with Mary, given the strain on him and on her. It is harder to predict what form his countertransference might take than it is in other scenarios. For example, he may be pulled in diametrically opposite directions, one moment identifying with Mary's depression, frustration, self-absorption, and the next moment resenting Mary as a demanding, depleting, parasitic woman. In addition to experiencing her as himself or as wife–mother, he may also experience her as his child, in need of reliable and loving fathering from him. Such rapid internal shifts may occur faster than he is able to bring them to his conscious awareness. On the surface, he may notice only that he is more tired than usual. If he can handle the fact that both of them have special needs in the present, and if he is able to seek and receive support for his needs elsewhere, then he may be available enough to actually understand Mary, empathize with her, enter into a therapeutic relationship with her, and focus on her psychotherapy. To the degree that his needs intrude into the dyad, he is at risk for reversing their roles and seeking healing from her. His own search for healing may include less than conscious wishes for succor, punishment, numbness, or sex.

The three examples of therapists represent countertransference pressures arising from the therapists' past history, present life, and characterological structure. They also indicate cross-gender tensions.

In response to the anxiety engendered by the treatment of a chronically ill person, therapists' defenses and countertransference scenarios are interwoven. These must be brought to awareness, clarified, and worked through in such a way that both therapist and patient may continue a therapeutic dialogue, free of hidden interfering anxieties and agendas. Countertransference issues may present themselves as anxieties, as affects, or as compensatory defensive reactions.

Common Countertransference Problems

In this section we give examples of therapists' countertransference reactions. We examine anxieties in general and body anxiety specifically. We look at affective countertransferences and defensive reactions.

Anxiety

Commonly experienced anxieties that are aroused in therapists by work with chronically ill patients revolve around death, failure, vulnerability, and loss. Death may be a possibility at any time, but, as we have noted throughout the book, some diseases pose quite certain and imminent threats to life. The intense work with dying patients often arouses fears about one's own death. One also may have fantasies about causing the patient's death. For example, a particular patient with heart disease was on the brink of death for 2 years before she actually died. Many times, she slipped close to death but rallied again and again before the end. The therapist worried frequently that she would inadvertently say something too intense for the patient to tolerate and, thus, precipitate the final crisis that would lead to the patient's demise. When the therapist became aware of this recurring anxiety, she realized that the patient also lived with the fear that some action on her part would precipitate death. Together, the therapist and the patient were able to talk about these fears and reduce the patient's anxiety substantially.

Fear of failure is another frequently encountered experience in work with chronically ill patients. Most psychotherapists are high achievers who want to help their patients become healthy. Many high achievers have a fear of failure rooted in early experiences of life. If this underlying anxiety goes unrecognized, a therapist can be drawn into a patient's intense or magical wishes for a cure, as happened to Michael's therapist in chapter 3. Propelled by a fear of failure, a therapist often offers suggestions and exhortations for treating the person's illness. In an often fruitless exercise, the therapist pushes the patient to spend limited energy and other resources that would be better spent on a more adaptive and preserving course.

Vulnerability is an omnipresent anxiety associated with chronic illness. Therapists may harbor anxiety about the disease itself or about symptoms they may share with their patients that may be minor or major. Therapists may be vulnerable also to their patients' great needs. Some people struggle with the burden of disease alone or in an environment with limited resources. Therapists may be the only source of support for patients in these circumstances. Unless therapists are aware of their vulnerability to being overwhelmed by patients' demands or needs, they risk acting in inappropriate ways. If therapists do not set adequate limits, they may actually become overwhelmed or "burned out." Alternatively, if they set overly stringent limits, they push the patient away from a needed resource and relationship. These two extremes occur more frequently than necessary in work with seriously and chronically ill patients, because therapists do not recognize the underlying anxiety, which is their vulnerability to becoming overwhelmed. Compassion fatigue takes its toll on caretakers in medicine, psychology, and the family alike.

Loss looms large in the work with all chronically ill patients. Apart from the special circumstance of death, patients' losses of functions, jobs, social status, even of reason bid therapists to recall their own losses in life. Awareness of therapist anxiety about loss can be managed and put to use therapeutically; lack of awareness can lead to depression or depressive reactions. Margaret was an 86-year-old woman with a brain tumor. She had been notably depressed and came to psychotherapy to discuss some issues about her life that were puzzling to her and that she wanted to resolve. She and her therapist worked together for 6 months, and Margaret reached the resolution she had been seeking. On the last day, Margaret declared that she had lived her life in the best way she could, and she left satisfied. The therapist was pleased that Margaret had achieved a sense of integrity and dignity. Later that day, Margaret abruptly lost her cognitive reasoning abilities; she died 5 weeks later.

For several months the therapist was unable to understand why she felt so sad: Margaret had finished what she set out to do and had reached the end of her long life comfortably. The therapist sought supervision and reviewed the case. Finally, she understood the relationship between her sadness about Margaret's death and her own anxiety about the loss of cognitive function. The therapist was shocked by Margaret's abrupt loss of cognitive function. She had anxious fantasies about losing her own ability to reason, the one faculty she most valued in herself.

Concern With Body

Offering psychotherapy to a patient with chronic physical illness carries some special challenges. It brings body awareness into the interaction, accompanied by the primitiveness of bodily needs, bodily functions, and bodily pains. Out of life history and experience, therapists develop attitudes toward their own bodies and toward others' bodies. They carry attitudes toward sickness, body functions, and disfigurement; toward sexual function and physical intimacy; toward taking care of others and being taken care of; and toward suffering. Like other people, therapists have fears about debilitation and decline, and most have had at least transitory terror about dying and about being left alone.

If therapists are not able to bring these universal, primitive, affective core sets to consciousness and integrate them, there is a substantial risk of becoming alienated from or overidentifying with the patient. However, if therapists can manage their particular body anxieties sufficiently, it is possible to remain engaged with the patients' process, rather than being pulled off into a defensive operation or becoming overwhelmed and subsumed by the patients' experiences.

Same-Sex Therapist and Patient

When the patient and therapist have many factors in common, the field is ripe for body anxiety and countertransference difficulties. The following vignette is based on such a set of difficulties and the resolution of the problem.

Nancy was a 50-year-old professional woman who was already in psychotherapy with Janet when she became ill with ovarian cancer. The course of surgery and subsequent chemotherapy led to a temporary suspension of psychotherapy. Nancy was away for several months because of complications stemming from her disease and treatment. Janet was aware that several months had passed beyond the expected hiatus, but she always found one reason or another for not calling and inquiring about how Nancy was doing. Eventually, Nancy called to ask for a session at the hospital, and Janet agreed.

Janet found herself very anxious about this particular visit, although she had conducted other psychotherapy sessions in the hospital from time to time. She stopped at the door and looked in. Nancy was bald and a fraction of her former weight. They began to talk and Nancy started to relate her events and experiences of the recent months. While Nancy talked, Janet began to experience strong body sensations of her own. She touched her own hair; her scalp felt strange. She had queasy abdominal feelings.

As Janet became aware of these bodily reactions, she began to realize why she had been so anxious about coming into the hospital and had postponed a call to Nancy. Janet was a woman in good health, also in her early 50s, who was just beginning to experience symptoms of menopause, a time of the cessation of ovarian function. Nancy's illness intensified Janet's existing feelings about loss of function. The devastating ovarian disease tapped into the wellspring of Janet's own fears about the vulnerability of her own changing body.

When Janet identified her personal issues of loss and vulnerability, she could understand how her previously unconscious anxieties about herself had inhibited her response to Nancy. The increased level of awareness of her own experience enabled Janet to listen and to be with Nancy. She was better able to facilitate Nancy's process of coping with the loss and vulnerability associated with ovarian cancer and its treatment.

Affects

Countertransferences are often experienced as affects. Several affectively related responses occur frequently during work with chronically ill patients. Anger is associated with frustration about the illness and the toll it exacts. Anger may also be a marker of frustration with patients who do not improve, who have no energy, or who do not fight pain well. In the messy domain of projection and projective identification, the therapist's anger may reflect the patient's anger, which he or she cannot express overtly or feel directly. Anger may mask other states, too, such as helplessness, with which most therapists must contend at times. In the case of Margaret's therapist, who felt sad and depressed, the persistent affective state of sadness provided the clue to the underlying anxiety about losing her cognitive function. As might be expected, the therapist's depressive constellation lifted shortly after she realized this.

When patients describe their illnesses in graphic detail, they may evoke feelings of distaste, disgust, or a wish to flee. These are common reactions in physicians, nurses, and psychotherapists, as well as the patients themselves and their family members. It is useful to find language for these affects, so they are not acted out. When the therapist is having a repulsion reaction, supervision or a consultation is indicated. Unacknowledged, these affects can destroy a psychotherapy and harm a patient. Understood, these affects can enhance a psychotherapy and move it forward, by enabling the patient to find language for his or her own feelings of disgust and distaste.

Positive affects such as hope and even euphoria can be clues to countertransference issues. A therapy can be infused with a sense of hope that comes from the therapist's wish for a cure. Everyone needs hope, but hope that arises from the therapist's need to succeed can blind him or her to the patient's need to deal with despair.

Most therapists who treat patients suffering from long-term illness discover a sense of helplessness that underlies the work. It may be only fleetingly present or there throughout the therapy. Helplessness is painful, and both therapist and patient struggle to find a sense of control. The acknowledgment of helplessness can be part of its resolution. Rarely is the helplessness complete. Most patients are able to discover some aspect of their life that is under their control. The avoidance of helplessness issues may result in struggles for control and the wasting of precious effort.

Defensive Reactions

Many defense mechanisms are used by therapists for protection against the anxieties and affects that accompany their work. These defenses hide the anxieties and affects associated with illness and disability, although they are not peculiar to working with a chronically ill population.

Denial functions as a primary defense. Therapists may not use total denial very often, but many deny either a partial reality or the severity of illness. The denial serves as a defense against helplessness. Therapists are quite capable of constructing a wall of denial, which is evident when they ignore information about the disease and assume a psychosomatic origin, which they believe they can cure. Most nonphysician psychotherapists know how to treat mental illness. Physical illness is another matter. It is easy to deny, especially when underlying body anxieties about death and helplessness exist. The choice to remain ignorant or dogmatic about illness and the situations surrounding illness prevents worries about vulnerability and loss from coming to light. The countertransference picture becomes even murkier when both physiological and psychological components drive the illness and a therapist or physician responds as if there were only one component.

Affects to illness can be dissociated and cut off. The therapist might perceive this phenomenon as a "spaciness," a time distortion, or it may become evident only through more intellectual channels. Affects can be defended against with isolation and intellectualization, as demonstrated in the countertransference example of Martin above. Martin also joined Mary in a collusion to "get on" with her life, before coming to grips with her painful feelings. Another method of avoiding a feeling is to act it out, which is an attempt to escape the experience of uncomfortable affects. Repression provides yet another method for the elimination of affects, that is, forgetting them.

Withdrawal from a patient may be expressed as boredom, a tendency to fall asleep, premature termination, cancellations of sessions, or extension of the intervals between sessions. Excuses are easy to find: The patient is too ill, needs time to rest, just came home from the hospital, is undergoing chemotherapy or dialysis. Janet used withdrawal to distance herself from Nancy and to keep her anxieties about her own body vulnerabilities hidden.

Identification or merger with a patient occurs with some regularity. The therapist may even have a fantasy in which he or she transfers health from the self to the patient.

Secular or religious moralizing, a dangerous defense against helplessness, is related to defensive omnipotence. The moralizing therapist conveys to the patient that if one has faith, then illness and its attendant problems will be overcome. If one changes lifestyle and does what is "good" and "correct," the disease will be reversed or halted. The harmful implication, of course, is that patients who do not get well are either sinners or deficient in some way. The moralizing therapist uses the stance to protect against uncertainty and the onslaughts of disease and death. There is an important distinction between a strong personal faith, which gives comfort and meaning to life, and a moralizing defense, which may be a countertransference reaction to illness.

The following are examples of signs that countertransference issues are prominent:

- The psychotherapy is not going well.
- The therapist is preoccupied with the patient out of session.
- The therapist's intense feelings persist.
- There is feedback from patient, supervisor, colleague, family, or friends regarding the therapist's preoccupation or intense feelings.

When signs of countertransference are present, self-analysis may clarify the underlying problem. Often, the therapist benefits from individual or peer-group supervision. Informal consultation with a trusted colleague is another avenue to understanding.

After the therapist has identified and clarified the countertransference issue, the knowledge can be used to benefit both patient and therapist. When Janet realized her anxiety about vulnerability related to her aging body, she addressed those issues privately. By gaining sufficient mastery within herself, she was able to help her patient, Nancy, articulate fears about ovarian cancer and come to terms with her vulnerability to pain and death.

In summary, good therapy demands awareness of anxieties, affects, and defenses; clarification of the meanings of these countertransference manifestations; and working through the problem to resolution. Practically speaking, it is not always possible to resolve countertransference issues in an ideal way. Nevertheless, it is realistic to aim for awareness and management of these responses.

7

Interaction: The Illness and the Patient's World

People with chronic illnesses interact with a world beyond their own bodies and personalities. Response to disease can be understood in terms of biology, psychology, sociology, and anthropology, as well as the philosophical perspective of time. For the clinician, it is necessary to take into account any special characteristics of the patient's milieu that may affect the psychological treatment. Special characteristics may be associated with personal, family, or social history; cultural diversity; role functions and values; the stigma of disease; life environment and resources; and life stages and transitions of time.

When outside factors impinge on someone's response to disease, a geometric progression of potential problems and risks may emerge. For the most part, however, clinicians may use the internal–external interaction as an opportunity to harness the strengths inherent in the patient's world. Good psychological evaluation and treatment planning identify both barriers and access to medical, psychological, and social support. Ignoring a patient's significant social and cultural experiences diminishes the likelihood of a successful psychotherapeutic outcome.

History

In addition to asking about a patient's medical history, practitioners should inquire about elements of a patient's background that are related to his or her body and attitudes toward it. A thorough history includes asking about previous illnesses in the patient and in family members or partners. It encompasses past ways of coping with those illnesses and the patient's interpretations of personal meaning surrounding the diseases. Patients who have a history of emotional, physical, and sexual abuse are at higher risk for poor coping with illness. They are at risk also for increased somaticizing as an indirect way of expressing pain, because it may be the only outlet for expression that is possible in their world. A history of alcohol or drug abuse complicates the picture further. The patient who no longer uses alcohol or drugs may be concerned about the dangers of addiction to pain medications. The patient who is currently dependent on alcohol or drugs often has poor judgment about disease management and responds to the added stressor of disease by increasing the substance usage patterns. The chemically dependent patient frequently has a dual diagnosis, intermingling substance-related problems with other mental health problems. Adding physical disease, whether it is exacerbated by the substance abuse or not, burdens the patient with a triple diagnosis.

The following case study provides an example of the importance of a physical history in the psychological treatment of the chronically ill patient. Gary, a 32-year-old affluent man with asthma, had been hospitalized for the condition with increasing frequency over a period of approximately 1 year. His physician referred him for psychological evaluation because his anxiety states seemed to be accelerating his physical deterioration. Gary had a history of alcoholism and cocaine abuse, which resulted in severe personal and social consequences (e.g., loss of his wife, job, driver's license, friends). With the assistance and structure of psychotherapy and Alcoholics Anonymous, he had been substance free for 6 years, and at the time of the referral, he was once again employed and had built a new social network. He was currently in a serious relationship with a stable woman. Gary grew up in a chaotic family system that was the source of much anxiety for him. His father had alcoholism, was violent toward his wife and children, and had sexually abused Gary's sister. His mother was psychotic and was often away from home for repeated hospitalizations. Gary was not in contact with his family.

Standard psychotherapeutic approaches and anxiety reduction support did not help alleviate Gary's intense fear of choking. As an alternative path to understanding how his history was affecting his responses and interactions with asthma, the consulting psychologist invited him to do a sand play. Sand play therapy is a Jungian approach that was originally developed and expanded in Europe (Kalff, 1980); it provides another way to enter the patient's world, a visual rather than a verbal manifestation of the self. It has been adapted by the author Carol Goodheart as a broad nonverbal technique, which may be similar to dreamwork for some patients or art therapy for others. Gary was given free reign to select any figures he wished from a display selection of hundreds of miniature figures of people, animals, mythic characters, vehicles for transportation, bridges, furniture, plants, stones, machines, and weapons. Wordlessly, he made his first selection, starting with a toilet, and created a scene in the sandbox. When he was finished, he was crying, and he told the story of the scene, which was the previously unexpressed experience of his early history. The scene itself was similar to a dream Gary had as a 14-year-old, during a crisis:

> A small boy is seated on the toilet. His arms and legs have been cut off. His genitals have been cut off and stuffed in his mouth. He is totally helpless and choking with fear. The woman looks on, but she does not help. The fat man with the whip is in control and he just smiles.

Gary's fear of choking was immediately relieved after that session. He understood how the anxiety of constricted airways during an asthma attack had become indistinguishable from his smothering and terrifying narrative of childhood. In subsequent sessions, the psychotherapy could build on his hard-won adult skills. He was able to challenge the old fear that he would be alone and no one would help him by counteracting the old script with his recent experiences of Alcoholics Anonymous, friends, and a medical team that responded to his needs. He went on to an improved regimen of self-care as well, managing the disease and his anxiety more effectively. He has not been rehospitalized for asthma. Uncovering his early history and understanding its meaning in the present was important to his psychotherapy and improved adaptation to the illness. The sand play was the therapeutic strategy used to help uncover the past.

Diversity

The need for sensitivity to the experience of others in a diverse society is a fundamental tenet of high-quality psychotherapy. People are grouped by race, gender, ethnicity, religion, sexual preference, age, intelligence, and socioeconomic status, as well as smaller subsets. They are also grouped by physical status, from the publicly acclaimed gifted athlete to the hidden, profoundly disabled person who is never seen by the general public.

In general, chronic disease lowers a person's social status, which, in turn, affects a person's self-esteem. Identification as a person with a chronic illness is added to other social identifications and groupings. A 45-year-old White, male, wealthy, married attorney with progressive coronary heart disease will have more health care options than a 19-year-old African American, unemployed, single mother with AIDS. Both have a compelling need for comprehensive medical and psychological services tailored to their specific capacities and resources. Unfortunately, differential societal attitudes toward their diseases and their other group identifications will hinder the AIDS patient's access to the best treatments.

Medically, women and minorities have been consistently underrepresented in clinical trials for disease treatments in the United States. Psychologically, women have less access to social support to cope with illness than do men, which may be associated with women's role as caregivers, leaving them adrift when they must change roles to become care receivers. Taylor and Aspinwall (1990) reported on several studies related to social support deficits that show disabled women are less likely than men to be or to get married (Kutner, 1987); women are more likely than men to be institutionalized, rather than cared for at home, after a stroke (Kelly-Hayes et al., 1988); unmarried women are likely to die sooner after a heart attack (Stern, Pascale, & Ackerman, 1977).

Audrey Lourde, a poet who died of breast cancer, was an African American and a lesbian. In *The Cancer Journals* (Lourde, 1980), she wrote movingly about the disjuncture that occurred when health care workers did not speak the language of her life experiences and concerns. Lesbians and gay men with chronic illnesses still struggle in many medical settings over such important issues as visitation by partners who are not considered family members by the hospital staff. They may face reactivated conflicts with family over such issues as giving durable power of attorney to the partner, rather than a family member.

Cultural and religious differences surrounding response to illness can be quite marked. Winifred was an elderly Jehovah's Witness with chronic inflammatory bowel disease. She had frequent episodes of intestinal bleeding that left her chronically anemic. On one occasion, she had extensive slow bleeding and her blood count dropped dangerously low. She agreed to hospital admission, but not to life-saving blood transfusions or to surgery. No interventions by physicians, social workers, or friends could persuade her to allow a transfusion, which would have been a violation of her religious principles. Winifred's bleeding stopped and she survived, although other patients have expired in such circumstances.

On the other hand, strong religious views can be especially supportive of medical treatment. We have been involved in the care of an African American adolescent with leukemia, who was hospitalized periodically with life-threatening crises. The boy's family belonged to a particular religious community. At times of crises, the family's minister came to "anoint" him. The act had a soothing effect on the teen and his family and may have facilitated his immune response. At first, the medical staff were reluctant to be present during the anointing ceremony, which involved a group joining of hands and prayers. However, intervening supportive work by a therapist allowed the physicians, nurses, family, and minister to form a team, which was much more effective in caring for the adolescent than individual staff members had been. As a result of this coalition, the parents were able to trust the medical staff and to communicate problems much earlier. Subsequently, there were fewer crises.

Mental or perceptual disability can have a major impact on response to physical disease. A mentally retarded person or a schizophrenic person may have difficulty communicating physical symptoms in a clear, understandable fashion. Other people may dismiss their complaints, attributing the complaints to their mental condition. Even a person with a less severe deficit may have difficulty. For example, an adolescent with dyslexia muddled through for 8 months with physical symptoms of postviral syndrome. His psychological pattern of self-doubt, combined with the awkward self-consciousness of his age, contributed to his lack of assertion. His condition remained unnoticed until he developed a major depression.

Role

Role shifts often occur with the onset and progression of chronic disease. People naturally grow into multiple roles over the course of life. Common adult roles include breadwinner, homework supervisor, emotional nurturer, disciplinarian, cook, chauffeur (family roles); worker, boss, team leader, troubleshooter, gofer, specialty expert, apprentice (work roles); church elder, charity volunteer, community leader, Little League coach, school board member (community roles). No one is ever truly prepared for the disruption of chronic illness and the role changes required to meet the challenges of managing an altered reality. The loss of a role represents a loss of power. It may signal also the loss of status, of competence, of contribution, of mastery. Sometimes, a role is not lost altogether but is scaled back or revised.

A new role arises with the advent of a chronic disease, the sick role. People use various styles to cope with, minimize, or maximize their role as sick people. However, the sick role calls on every patient to comply (with disease-controlling or health-promoting regimens) and to depend on others (to a greater or lesser extent, depending on the disease and its progression).

As individuals adapt to changes in physical functioning, they alter participation in their everyday roles. Heightened needs for privacy or pain management, for example, pull the patient away from former levels of involvement with the outside world. Lowered self-esteem, depression, pain, and shame about body disfigurement may all contribute to a decrease in sexual functioning. A couple who have been accustomed to a comfortable sense of themselves as adult lovers and financial contributors to their household will be under severe strain if one partner can no longer participate sexually and financially. Their roles may shift from adult–adult to adult–child to parent–child. There is no magic map to guide the psychological transition from independent adult functioning to appropriate levels of dependence for the level of disability. Coping with a chronic illness as it changes and progresses is a changing and progressive process for patients and their families. Psychological interventions are most effective if they are grounded in this fluidity of illness progressions.

Because the needs of the sick person do not remit (and often increase), the role of primary caretaker to the patient is a demanding one. Caretaker family members are subject to role fatigue and burnout (Goldstein, Regnery, & Wellin, 1981). In some instances, it is the emotional press, rather than the physical demands, that overtaxes the caregiver. We have treated women in the past year who sought psychological services to better deal with their chronically ill husbands' tempers and rages. In three of the four cases, the ill husbands controlled their tempers with others and lost control only with their spouses. In the fourth case, the ill husband (a young man with an incurable cancer) was rageful and abusive toward his children, relatives, and neighbors.

Stigma

The *American Heritage College Dictionary* (3rd ed.; Houghton Mifflin, 1993) defines *stigma* as "a mark or token of infamy, disgrace, or reproach." Much of the world views sick and disabled people as abnormal, "less than," unacceptable, and at fault for their own predicaments. Falvo (1991) observed that anxiety-provoking and threatening conditions heighten the likelihood of stigma becoming attached to those conditions. Public policy about illness and disability (from the lepers of ancient times to the AIDS patients of today) has been shaped by the tensions between advocates for humane medical and social responsiveness and a frightened populace trying to distance themselves from anxiety by ostracizing the victim. Although many health care and mental health care professionals are dedicated advocates for the chronically ill, any of us may harbor prejudicial distancing attitudes toward conditions that arouse our personal anxieties.

Discrimination is a fact of life for people with chronic conditions, in practical terms like job rejection and health insurance rejection. Even a cancer survivor who has been disease free for 10 or more years and who has no physical impediments may be turned down for jobs and insurance. Despite statutory governmental protections (e.g., the Americans With Disabilities Act), discrimination remains commonplace in the stories of the patients we treat. Summaries of cancer survivors' rights and redress procedures are provided in pamphlets that are made available by the American Cancer Society (1993) and Candlelighters Childhood Cancer Foundation (1993).

Stigma interacts with self in a potentially debilitating way. It has an impact on self-identity and self-esteem and on conscious and unconscious expectations of object relations. In "Illness, Stigma, and AIDS," Herek (1990) stated that "in general, a stigma is most extensively incorporated into the self-concept when it generates extreme and consistent negative reactions on the part of others" (p. 132). He identified several coping strategies used by stigmatized group members to preserve self-esteem: the attribution of negative social experiences to external stigma and positive social experiences to internal personal qualities; the devaluation of qualities no longer possessed; and the selection of stigmatized others for social comparison. The use of these strategies would seem to demonstrate adaptive progress toward a reconsolidated self in a changed personal world.

Visible disfigurement elicits negative social responses that are hurtful and may shape future willingness to go out in public and enter into new social situations. For example, a friend of one of the authors is a 72-year-old woman with severe rheumatoid arthritis. The visible signs of her arthritis are present but not unusual. Her remarkable physical feature is highly blemished skin, which is the result of chronic bleeding under the skin, a side effect of steroid medication for the disease. This bright, pleasant woman had been physically and socially active, despite significant disability, until she was emotionally wounded by an upsetting social experience. It took months to regain her personal and social equilibrium.

The stigmatizing event occurred at a club swimming pool, where the woman had been swimming regularly for several years. She swam for physical therapy and for the pleasure and exercise. One day, an onlooker was offended by the appearance of her skin and attributed it to "open sores, some kind of disease, or God knows what else." The onlooker did not speak to the woman with arthritis, but instead enlisted the support of others and spoke to the pool manager. The pool manager told her about the member's concern with some embarrassment and asked her not to swim there anymore. He couched his request as a statement about her comfort. Although the woman continues an active life, she has a residual body embarrassment that has not resolved with time. She will not expose her body in a bathing suit or swim in anyone's presence, including immediate family members at a private family pool. She has managed the arthritis very well for many years but is still struggling with feelings about the appearance of her skin.

Environment

Given the importance of social support for people with chronic physical conditions, we try to assess the strengths and limitations in the patient's environment. The family system, medical system, employment system, and socioeconomic system seem to be the key environmental factors related to the patient's need for external resources. Strengths in one area can sometimes be enhanced to offset deficits in another system.

A family member is most frequently, but not always, the primary caregiver and support person for the ill patient. It is also beneficial if other family members are involved and contribute to the support and tasks as they evolve. Because not all family members can contribute in the same ways, they should be involved in the functions they do best and are not likely to shirk out of anxiety or resentment. If the illness progresses and disability becomes great, the strains on a family grow proportionately also. Power et al. (1988) recommended respite care as a resource for families of the seriously ill, based on the following principles:

- No one is completely prepared for illness or disability.
- Illness changes a family and challenges its resources.
- The illness process brings out the best and worst in families.
- Disability can deplete family resources as well as create them.
- Often the only support is family.
- All people do not have families they can rely on.
- Not all families are capable of responding to the illness and disability of a family member.
- New skills are needed by the family to meet the new challenges created by illness.
- Coping with chronic disability is an ongoing developmental process for the patient as well as the family.
- Existing health care resources can help as well as hinder adjustment.
- Respite care is often the difference between coping and deteriorating. (p. 279)

The medical system can function as a powerful source of support in a patient's life. It can function also as a frustrater, confuser, controller, or ignorer. In general, there are enough choices in most medical systems for patients to find avenues of collaboration and responsiveness. Hospitals have ombudspersons or offices of social service that are useful for most patients. Sometimes, psychological interventions are geared to helping patients make better use of the medical system components that are available to them. For example, some patients must learn what questions to ask. Questions from the Medical Template can be useful (see p. 16). Some patients need help with framing their concerns in a way that increases the likelihood of a useful response. Other helpful interventions include communication skills, assertion skills, and organization skills training.

The employment system is central to many people's sense of worth and identity. It may constitute their only financial security. The likelihood of employer accommodations for a chronically ill person is dependent on the specific needs of the person and the capacities of the setting. Many patients need time flexibility for brief periods (such as an afternoon physician or physical therapy appointment) or over time (for periods of disability when the patient is unable to work). Others try not to take time off. They go to work despite discomfort and fatigue, because they need the income. They may be fearful of losing a job for repeated absences. Self-employed people are even more vulnerable, if they cannot sustain their businesses through a chronic illness. Referrals to human services departments in the employment setting or to community and religious organizations' social services may be warranted.

A patient's place in the socioeconomic system affects all the other systems referred to above. The chronically ill person with a surplus of financial resources can afford to hire household help to ease the family's strain, can afford choices among medical providers and systems, and can afford to work fewer hours or not at all. However, only a tiny minority of people have the financial resources to sustain themselves and their families without worrying about their financial future. Therefore, practitioners must be aware of patients' realistic financial anxieties and facilitate their educative process to discover alternative sources of financial assistance whenever possible. An effective means of obtaining financial assistance information is to contact the national organization for a particular disease (e.g., cancer patients may contact the American Cancer Society). Help with transportation and the cost of equipment can often be obtained (see chapter 11). At the local level, hospital ombudspersons and social service personnel also may be helpful with financial assistance.

Life Stage and the Social Meaning of Time

Concepts related to body change and psychological change are embedded throughout the book. People pass through physical and psychological stages of development across the life span. In addition, they pass through stages of development across the span of their illnesses. The purpose in introducing the interaction between time and the world's response is to underscore the disjuncture between the changing needs of the patient and the fixed responses they often receive.

For example, it is routinely expected that elderly people with chronic conditions will withdraw from the world, be fretful, decrease activities, and suffer from poor concentration. In a younger person, those symptoms are more likely to be noted by a physician as a constellation of worry, anxiety, and depression that should be treated. The elderly patient needs comprehensive psychological and medical treatment as much as the younger person does. Treatment should include the depression and work on the contributing factors and ongoing quality-of-life needs as well.

At the other end of the age spectrum, seriously ill babies and children touch a primal chord in most adults. The threat to a child's life arouses profound empathy because of the magnitude of the loss in a life that people believe has not yet been lived. Children represent the future—of a society, of a community, and of a family. Children with a progressive fatal disease have very special needs, as do their families. People often treat a sick child as fragile, regardless of his or her present capacities. They have difficulty allowing sick children to be as "normal" as they are striving to be (e.g., eating junk food and engaging in horseplay with other children when they feel up to it). When children are in a final transitional stage and nearing death, many people withdraw from them and their surrounding family members, either because they do not believe they can tolerate experiencing the death of children or because they are afraid they cannot offer anything of value to the children or their families. Paradoxically, seriously ill children and their families need external support both to help them hold on to the ordinariness of life for as long as they can and, when the time comes, to let go of an extraordinary life.

Summary

The special characteristics of patients' backgrounds and milieus have been introduced to further the understanding of responses to disease and its treatment. In this chapter, the importance of personal, family, and social history; cultural and religious diversity; and changes in role functions and values have been discussed. The stigma of disease, the life environment, and available resources have been noted. Finally, developmental life stages and the social meaning of time have been explored. In chapters 8 and 9, these factors are further explored with respect to children and families.

8

Children With Chronic Illness

Practitioners must realize that psychological interventions with children and adolescents are different from those used with adults. Much of the material in earlier chapters is relevant to chronically ill children and their families (e.g., the acquisition of medical information, the use of the templates, the understanding of temperament and personality organization). However, there is an essential difference in the treatment model that has importance for the underpinnings of effective psychological treatment. For chronically ill adults, the focus is on reconsolidation after the disorganization of an established sense of self. The task emphasis shifts for children, who have a developing self that has not yet achieved a mature identity. The goal with children is to foster a sense of safety, security, regularity, and predictability of life so that natural growth and healthy development of the self can occur.

The child with a chronic illness has been robbed of the "invulnerable self" expectation, a crucial part of growing up. Sick children often have to face the multiple losses, pains, and limitations that are more common to aging adults. How does someone prepare a child to carry on a satisfactory adult life with a history of living with illness for his or her first 15 to 20 years? Beyond day to day managing and survival, living with an uncertain physical reality requires a stable internal psychological structure of a self. A certain amount of denial of anxiety and of insistence on "normalcy" fosters successful adaptation to chronic illness in children. A literature review by Whitt (1984) supports this view on adaptive denial. Children who make use of these adaptive strategies seem to regain a measure of invulnerability.

Multiple Approaches for Multiple Problems When Treating Young Children

Approximately 30% of children in the United States have a chronic disease (Meyer & Lewis, 1994). The 1988 National Health Interview Survey (Newacheck & Taylor, 1992) estimated that 65% of these chronic conditions were mild, 30% were moderately severe and involved disabilities, and 5% were severe. Some of these childhood diseases will continue into adulthood, such as asthma, diabetes, seizure disorders, sickle cell anemia, cystic fibrosis, and heart disease. Some diseases will be cured, in remission, or "outgrown," such as juvenile rheumatoid arthritis, cancer, and some asthmas. Some diseases will recur or flare acutely, such as some cancers. Some diseases may shorten the life span or may result in death before adulthood is reached, such as cystic fibrosis, muscular dystrophy, Down's syndrome, or the ataxias.

Children with chronic diseases may grow to adulthood with residual psychological scars caused by the pain and trauma they have experienced, and they may come to consider their relationship with a crisis team to be the norm for all relationships. Under duress children may form lifelong structures based on avoiding tasks because of pain or disability (a conscious or preconscious choice), using the illness for secondary gain (an unconscious choice), or developing somaticizing overlays to physical attunement (an unconscious choice). Such tactics can be developmentally crippling. Psychological intervention, both prevention and remediation, can help children and their families to integrate better the responses to disease with the maturational tasks of life.

There is no clear dividing line between individual and family psychotherapy, because the treatment of ill children involves special work with the parents. Usually, parents are given the medical information and bear the responsibility for decisions and for caretaking. Parents of very young children bear the entire burden, whereas parents of adolescents share the knowledge and the choices with the teen, who often is given information directly by the medical team. Conflicts can and do erupt between children and parents over treatment compliance issues, especially when children reach adolescence. Psychotherapy may involve siblings or other extended family members as well, depending on their needs. Siblings of chronically ill children reverberate to the jagged patterns of crisis and limitation in the household with their own range of responses. These include envy, resentment, jealousy, guilt, anxiety, identification, craving for a "normal" family, demands for attention, depression, impulsive behavior, denial, empathy, caring, and compensatory reaction formations against negative emotions in such forms as martyrdom or exaggerated altruism. The dynamic meaning of the illness for the family members and their handling of the sick child has a life-shaping impact on the child's psychological development.

Often, there is no clear dividing line between prevention and remediation in psychological treatment either. As a rule of thumb, the coping and the adaptation models tend to fall more toward the prevention end of the treatment continuum and the trauma models of treatment more toward the remediation end. In practical terms, this means that elements of both are used in the dynamic focus on the development of a stable self.

A developmental approach takes into account the life stage of the child. Particular attention is paid to the activities that make up the life tasks to be accomplished or navigated during the period. Sutkin (1984) observed that a disabling condition obstructs normal activity appropriate to the life stage. As a consequence, the disruption to development is associated with a lack of the "essential qualities required for a healthy and complete ego" (p. 2). Unfortunately, children with chronic physical disorders are at risk for psychological disorders, if their natural growth trajectories are thwarted and if they are unable to find adaptive alternative paths. The guiding principle of the fostering of a child's growth toward a stable adult self is commensurate with a developmental perspective on psychological treatment.

In the following sections, we discuss trauma resolution in children with cancer, a coping paradigm in connection with diabetic children, and the stage of adolescence to highlight a developmental emphasis. The selection of a treatment approach depends more on the child than on the disease. For example, some children with cancer need a coping approach; for them, a trauma resolution approach would not be appropriate. It is not our intent to limit treatment choices to the particular match-ups presented here for illustration. To the contrary, this discussion is intended to convey a hint of the variety of clinical resources that are available.

Cancer

Treatment and aftermath.   Children who are cancer veterans and their families comprise a special population for whom community psychological services are scarce once they leave active medical treatment. Not too many years ago, a diagnosis of childhood cancer was a death sentence, whereas now it is considered a chronic disease to be managed over time. Survival rates give cause for hope, and many infants and children with cancer grow up to be healthy adults. The treatment for many childhood cancers is aggressive, however, in a way unknown even a generation ago, and these treatments engender side effects that are very difficult for a child to endure. After treatment there remains the likelihood of late effects, the consequences of radiation therapy and chemotherapy. It has been said often that a life-threatening cancer hits the whole family, not merely one individual. At no time is that more true than when the patient is a child, because the child is dependent on parents for all of the decisions and the caretaking needed, and child carries the family's hopes for the future.

There are multiple levels of stress for these cancer families (as is true also for families with other diseases). Acute stress occurs during active illness and frightening, painful treatments. Afterward, chronic stress continues for families: There is pain if the disease is progressive and uncontrollable; there is anxiety even when the treatment ends successfully because of fears of a recurrence; and there is the strain and worry of coping with the long-term sequelae of the treatments given, that is, residual physical and/or mental disabilities.

Children undergoing active cancer treatments are assaulted by physical intrusion—surgeries, amputations, chemotherapy, radiation therapy, bone marrow aspirations, nasogastric tube insertions, placement of ports or broviacs (lines for medicines or blood that are sutured into a major blood vessel in the chest). Not surprisingly, these children look like acute trauma victims. Very few psychotherapists in the general practice community see the children or their families during this time. If available, psychological support is provided by the hospital treatment team.

What happens when the treatment ends and the families try to resume their lives after the acute crisis phase? It is essential that they master and work through the trauma. Stuber, Christakis, Housekamp, and Kazak (1996) reported the following research findings (based on responses to their Post Traumatic Stress Disorder Reaction Index):

1. Most survivors of childhood malignancies are doing well psychologically 2 years posttreatment.

2. A significant proportion of the children (12.5%) report symptoms consistent with a severe level of posttraumatic stress (e.g., bad dreams, fearful thoughts about cancer, nervousness).

3. A high percentage of the mothers (39.7%) and the fathers (33.3%) suffered from severe posttraumatic symptoms (anxiety about relapse, upset feeling states when thinking of cancer, reexperiencing disturbing scenes).

Primary clinicians may be able to apply an understanding of a psychological perspective to the resolution of trauma so that the individual and the family can bring the best possible coping responses to bear on continuing physical problems. Cancer families should have the benefit of psychological assistance routinely, to work through the trauma experience, without a diagnosis of mental illness. They carry the posttraumatic stress response pattern within them, even if they do not show outward signs of dysfunction and seem to carry their burden courageously. "Normal" people in abnormal circumstances require both psychological and medical expertise. Unfortunately, such care is far from the norm.

Questions parents frequently ask. The psychotherapist can help parents anticipate some of the particularly stressful situations surrounding medical treatment and illness and plan for ways to move through those times. Practical examples include the following dilemmas:

Should I hold my young child while the procedure is being done? Is that a positive gesture, or will the child feel betrayed by the parent? In general, most parents (usually the mother, but not always) opt to stay with the child. Parents with children in active cancer treatment tell us they stay and hold the child's hand or stroke the forehead or talk reassuringly, even when they themselves are scared or upset, because they do not want the child to have to suffer alone. Such a choice communicates the message that the experience can be borne successfully, if parents are able to control their own anxiety sufficiently to facilitate the child's experience. Redd (1990, p. 575) has identified two distinctive parental response patterns correlated with high distress levels in children: extreme emotional reactivity and the more subtle scenario of too much support, which leads to compliance with the child's every demand of the child and fuels his or her fears. In such cases, the child may do better without the parents present, and some older children even ask parents to leave the room. In that event, parents need help to remain supportive in other ways.

Parents should not be responsible for restraining the child, however, and we believe that both parent and child can differentiate emotionally between holding and restraint. The parents who choose to remain present while their children undergo painful procedures also act as monitors and advocates for their children. They insist on time outs, if feasible; on better pain medication or sedation management, if necessary; and on more experienced medical personnel to handle the procedure more humanely and efficiently, if warranted.

How can I help my child not to be anxiously awaiting pain and intrusion all the time? The anxiety cannot be removed entirely, but it can be reduced. One strategy is to keep uncomfortable procedures away from the daily routine. For example, a child's bed or crib should never be used as the site for procedures, but should be kept as a safe place. This choice is an important one, whether the bed is at home or in the hospital. Other strategies include giving the child something else to be involved with and think about in life besides the cancer treatment, and giving the child new ways to cope.

How can I help my child cope with the painful or dreaded procedure? Many children struggle with anticipatory anxiety, nausea, and vomiting as chemotherapy time approaches. Bone marrow aspirations and other procedures cause anxiety and immediate pain and distress. Families can work with cancer center staff to ensure that both parents and children are given coping strategies appropriate to the situation. Practical tools that have been beneficial include positive motivation (incentives as opposed to punishment, which is never beneficial), distraction and focusing techniques such as hypnosis to engage the attention elsewhere and reduce the intensity of distress, and breathing exercises to decrease arousal that escalates anxiety and codes fear. (For a comprehensive discussion of these and many other strategies and techniques, see Redd, 1990, "Behavioral Interventions to Reduce Child Distress.") Parents and children tell us these techniques do work, but to varying degrees, depending on the severity of the procedures and the resources of the child. The art lies in devising and adapting techniques that the child is able to incorporate and use successfully.

My 5-year-old is acting like a baby again. She is asking to be fed since the baby has been sick. What should I do? This is a prime example of sibling regression as a response to a family crisis. Clinicians can guide the parents to understand the regression as normal, to feed the little girl and go along with her for a bit until the equally normal push to move forward developmentally resumes, perhaps with some parental encouragement.

How can I follow the recommended guidelines for nutritious food intake during my child's chemotherapy, when he cannot seem to eat anything? Many parents seem to feel guilty and frustrated about their child's diet. The ones who do best seem to focus on the reality of what is possible, rather than the ideal. For example, one mother told us that she was so pleased for her son when he could eat something, she was willing to go shopping at midnight to get licorice for him if that would suffice. Another mother told us her 13-month-old baby ate only Cheetos (in addition to breast milk) for 3 months. At one point, when the extended family had a celebration for another relative, four different relatives brought bags of Cheetos for this baby. Both of the families mentioned in this example were aware of normal nutritional needs, but they were responsive first to the capacities of their children.

What can I do when no one seems to have an answer to this problem (whatever it is)? The best answer seems to be to keep trying and to look for partial solutions, not magic. Sometimes, relatively simple approaches offer some relief. For example, the Cheetos baby mentioned above developed a severe burn reaction that covered her entire diaper area, in a possibly idiosyncratic response to a chemotherapy drug secreted through the urine. In intense pain, the baby was hospitalized and given significant doses of morphine to control the pain. None of the physicians knew why the reaction was occurring. The mother and grandmother, however, were primarily concerned with how to obtain relief for the baby's pain, so they talked to everyone they came in contact with at the hospital, including other parents and medical personnel from departments other than the oncology unit. A radiation unit nurse mentioned the use of Domeboro Solution, which she said had been applied to elderly radiation patients with some success. The physicians were skeptical but said it would be harmless to try. Within 5 minutes of the first soak in the Domeboro Solution, the baby was temporarily relieved. Thereafter, the treatment was used routinely, along with antibiotic and antifungal medications, until the condition was resolved. When the issue is comfort, not cure, there is always another avenue to try, always room for improvement.

Everyone in the family seems to have a short temper; what can I do about all this anger? Anger is frequently a by-product of frustration, pain, loss, and trauma. It is also a response to anxiety in some people. Clinicians can help parents understand it as a natural phenomenon and respond to it better in themselves, in the child with the chronic illness, and in the siblings. Parents can be guided toward individual plans that include (a) allowance for expression that is contained within nondestructive limits (e.g., a 4-year-old might need a punching doll, a 34-year-old might need a 20-minute walk to regain composure); (b) response to the pressing need that triggered the outburst (e.g., the primary caretaker needs a respite from caretaking, the ill child needs another satisfying activity to replace the one no longer available); (c) tolerance for the legitimacy of angry feelings (e.g., "I know you're mad. You have every right to be disappointed and grumpy today, but you may not hit me. Instead, you can talk to me about it, or we can do something else—maybe work on your model airplane—or you can spend some time alone if that feels better right now."); and (d) channeling the aggression of anger into a positive fighting spirit to handle the traumatic and wearing circumstances (e.g., we overheard one child complaining to another about being afraid of someone at the hospital, and the other youngster replied, "Well, the bestest thing is to pretend you're a Power Ranger—then you're the strongest one and can zap 'em if you have to.").

What can I do to help my child face returning to school during treatment and after treatment? The goal in this instance is to facilitate the child's transition back into the school setting. The American Cancer Society and many cancer treatment centers have special programs for this purpose. They offer programs to educate teachers about what to expect when the child reenters the class. Specific cancer centers also offer speakers who will go into a child's class before reentry and educate the children about very practical matters, such as why the child is bald (chemotherapy), or has a puffy face (steroids), or has a tube in his or her nose (feeding tube) or chest (for blood or chemotherapy). Such programs make life easier for the child with cancer and for the classmates, because what they imagine is often worse than the reality. Classmates respond better and are less anxious when they are given the information they need to allay their fears. They are less likely to reject and stigmatize the child who looks different if they can understand the differences at their own maturational level of development. Where such programs are not available, a parent may schedule a conference with the teacher and provide information about the child's needs and condition. Parents who are knowledgeable might speak to the class as well as with the teacher. Candlelighters (see the resources listed in chapter 11), a national organization for children with cancer and their families, can serve as a resource to identify helpful professionals, volunteers, and programs throughout the country. For example,

Candlelighters provides educational materials on the special learning needs of children who have learning problems after cranial irradiation (e.g., for leukemias, brain tumors) and some chemotherapy drugs. These children have a legal right to an individualized educational plan, but many schools do not offer it unless parents request it. Candlelighters serves as a clearinghouse for many other services and sources of information as well, such as handling medical and adjunctive reimbursement problems with insurers and managed care organizations

How are we ever going to get through this? The clinician can explore the individual and family needs and tailor an individual program, but it is particularly useful to facilitate the family's access to community resources and supportive network possibilities beyond the family. For example, support groups for parents and for children with cancer, both age specific and disease specific, are offered in many parts of the country. Camps for cancer children and families give opportunities for a proactive response to illness and the sharing and receiving of information, common experiences, coping, and hope. Sometimes parents must try more than one group before they find one that fulfills their needs. One mother whose child was newly diagnosed with cancer attended a group offered by the hospital oncology unit but found the other mothers there all had children in the terminal stages of cancer. She continued her search until she found a group of mothers comparable to herself. Another couple (mother and father) went to a group whose leader offered no structure or leadership in focusing the discussion, so they moved on to another group. Adolescents often respond to group support because they are especially peer-oriented at that stage of their lives.

Posttraumatic Stress Disorder

Pynoos (1990) identified seven categories of extreme stressors that have been associated with posttraumatic stress disorder (PTSD) in children, one of which is the occurrence of life-threatening illness and life-endangering medical procedures. PTSD in children is similar to PTSD in adults, but there are important differences related to age and developmental level. Pynoos developed PTSD criteria for children over the age of 3 that are similar to adult criteria:

- the experience of an event as distressing that anyone would consider distressing,
- the reexperiencing of the event repeatedly in various ways,
- response symptoms of numbing, avoidance, and increased arousal.

For children younger than 3 years, Drell, Siegel, and Gaensbauer (1993, p. 293) described PTSD as "a lasting dysfunction in intra- or interpersonal life that follows from and is related to overwhelming experience(s)." They reported that infants and toddlers may have both a broader and a narrower range of reaction than the older person, based on capacities for organizing experience perceptually, globally, and creating memory for relations between perceptual experiences. After a thorough review of the literature, they concluded that "the capacity for perceiving and remembering events, including traumatic ones, clearly exists from the earliest months of life" (p. 293). They proposed (p. 295) an additive system of trauma symptom categorization for these infants as follows:

- Age 0–6 months: Hypervigilance; exaggerated startle; dysregulation; irritability or withdrawal.
- Age 6–12 months: Any of the above; marked anxiety in strange situations; more specific anger in particular situations; more active attempts to avoid specific situations as mobility increases; developmental regressions; sleep disorders/night terrors.
- Age 12–18 months: Any of the above; "clinginess" with caregivers; avoidance of particular affects or situations that evoke the affects; over or under usage of words associated with the trauma.
- Age 18–24 months: Any of the above; preoccupation with symbols of the trauma; nightmares; more enlarged verbal preoccupations.
- Age 24–36 months: Any of the above; symptoms as in older children.

As children grow, they move from total dependence on caregivers to provide stimulus barriers (so they will not become overwhelmed by auditory, visual, or tactile experiences) to development of their own ability to regulate experience physiologically and psychologically. Therefore, the treatment for childhood PTSD would seem to need tailoring according to the child's ability (a) to manage the disturbing stimuli originally and (b) to incorporate the experience over time, without lasting dysfunction.

When an infant undergoes an upsetting event, commonsense interventions include physical soothing, rocking, crooning, stroking, and enabling sucking (pacifier or fingers). This helps physiological regulation, and it quickly moves the baby from a distressing experience to a pleasurable and reassuring one. Most parents do this automatically and naturally, but on occasion parents are so traumatized by the event that they freeze and do nothing, or they are so overwhelmed by their own emotions that they cannot respond to the child. Babies, toddlers, and children all need caretakers who allow them to react to the trauma and who communicate by their own responsiveness that those reactions are manageable. The greatest gift a psychotherapist can give to a traumatized child may be to help the parents move from an overwhelmed state to an appropriately responsive one. In addition to needing soothing, toddlers can respond to talk about the event and may benefit from it even before they themselves are able to put their experience into words. Older children usually respond well to talk about troubling experiences, and they turn actively to trusted caregivers for help when distressed by painful stimuli. Children are capable of expressing anger at any age, from infancy on up. Their anger may be expressed as a total body experience of tension and crying, yelling, throwing things, threatening to run away or retaliate, saying "I hate you," and the like. Anger is a natural response to the experience of being provoked, and medical procedures can be highly provocative.

At a bare minimum, children who undergo a potentially traumatic experience need soothing, time to recover from a hurtful or frightening procedure, opportunities for distraction and another focus (to help with the process of managing the experience), and outlets afterward for aggressive responses and large motor activities (e.g., pounding, kicking, swooping play). Children need encouragement and praise for attempts to manage (e.g., holding still and counting), not for mastery of anxiety reduction.

The psychological assessment of the aftereffects of trauma on a child requires a careful history taken from the parents. The evaluation must take into account the developmental stage at the time of the illness onset and the traumatic medical treatment, the concomitant events and interventions, and the symptoms and residual effects. One must evaluate also the parents' reactions to the trauma, responsive capacities, and needs for support, education, or treatment.

The psychological treatment of children with PTSD and their families is based on the therapeutic goal of helping the children master the trauma through repeatedly reexperiencing the trauma and its meaning, in tolerable affective doses, in a safe setting. Children need structured play and play materials to recreate and communicate the trauma. To integrate the strong feelings aroused by the trauma, they need empathy and an "emotional container" provided by the setting, the increasing distance of time from the event, and the person of the therapist. They need time to make "sense" of what has happened to them. When parents participate in therapeutic sessions, there is an added set of benefits. Drell et al. (1993) believed the parents' presence facilitates their own understanding of the child's internalization of the trauma, encourages them to appreciate and support the psychotherapeutic treatment process, models communication about feelings that can enhance the parent–child interactions at home, and allows them to receive support from the therapist as their own reactions and responses are stirred by the process. Additionally, involved parents are often able to be more supportive and less frightened if the child's symptoms become heightened during the period when the child is remembering and grappling with feelings associated with the traumatic illness.

Diabetes: Stress, Coping, Adaptation

Practitioners who want to help children and their families meet the challenges of living with diabetes must understand the basics and the never-ending adjustments required by the condition. Diabetes is a complex condition, characterized by hyperglycemia (chronic high blood sugar). In type I insulin-dependent diabetes mellitus, the body secretes little or no insulin, a necessary substance for the metabolism of glucose. A body unable to use glucose must turn to fat for fuel, a process that produces ketones as a by-product and leads to diabetic ketoacidosis, an acute condition that results in death if it remains untreated. Historically, this was known commonly as juvenile onset diabetes. Another form of later onset diabetes, occurring in adults typically over the age of 40, is non–insulin-dependent diabetes mellitus (type II). The physical symptoms are thirst, frequent urination, and weight loss. The medical treatment goal is to reach and maintain stable blood glucose levels that are within normal range.

Czyzewski (1988, pp. 270–271) described the regimen necessary to manage type I diabetes. Children and their families must come to terms with the constraints. Reduced to its basic elements, the regimen includes the following:

1. Take one or more insulin injections daily.

2. Time meals to coincide with insulin action.

3. Balance amount of carbohydrates eaten with amount of insulin injected to metabolize the carbohydrates.

4. Monitor blood glucose several times daily (fingertip prick for blood drop, place on reagent strip, time reaction, read results). If high, test urine for ketones.

5. Give additional insulin for high glucose level.

6. Exercise routinely for facilitation of insulin action and balance with insulin intake.

7. Readjust insulin needs when physical illness or upset triggers hormonal reactions that increase glucose levels.

Diabetic children and families have both acute and chronic periods of stress, as discussed in regard to children with cancer, but the rhythms of their condition and opportunities for growing self-management are different. Newly diagnosed children and their families have many new practical skills to master, as well as the emotional work of assimilation of an altered lifestyle due to disease. Experienced children and families have periods of volatility too, because not even ironclad attempts at rigid control will guarantee physiological stasis. Although many children attain a comfortable adaptation, the psychological strain stemming from the diabetic management routines, challenges, and disappointments is significant for a sizable subset of children, as indicated by the estimates of nonadherence to medical treatment protocols. Compliance levels in chronic disease treatments average only 50% across the board among children, adolescents, and adults, with a range between 10% and 80% in children; adolescents show poorer compliance as a group, with rates between only 40% and 55% (Hymovich & Hagopian, 1992).

Chronically ill people, including children, modify coping efforts in multidimensional ways throughout the course of an illness. Justice (1988) described coping with chronic disease as a cycle, in which people pass through many steps and stages as they try to handle a problem. That perspective seems particularly relevant to the psychological treatment of diabetic children and families, as they pass through multiple stages of both coping and "normal" development. Diabetes does not present a discrete problem, but rather a universe of problems to be handled. Murphy's (1974) work on vulnerability and resilience in children framed coping as a process involving attempts and efforts at mastery over potentially threatening, challenging, or gratifying situations.

Treatment within a coping paradigm. Wertlieb, Jacobson, and Hauser (1990, p. 73) presented a comprehensive stress and coping paradigm to understand child and family adaptation to insulin-dependent diabetes mellitus. Their model illustrates the interrelated cause-and-effect relationships among the following factors:

- stress origins (developmental, major life event, hassles, chronic);
- coping processes (adherence, knowledge/skills, emotion management);
- resources/moderators (social support, self-esteem, health beliefs, ego development, temperament);
- outcomes (metabolic control, complications, behavior symptoms, adjustment).

Their thoughtful review of the research literature offers a set of resources that can be used as one starting point for the evaluation and treatment of chronically ill children. The coping framework may be adapted also to other chronic conditions (e.g., asthma, juvenile rheumatoid arthritis), just as the trauma model is applicable to a wider range of conditions than cancer treatments. The experienced practitioner may wish to extrapolate particular aspects from the material and integrate the relevant parts into a personalized treatment orientation. The following summary is adapted from Wertlieb et al. (1990, pp. 79–94):

Coping Processes (identified by Kovacs & Feinberg, 1982) used by the diabetic children and their parents to manage negative affective problems (e.g., anger, depression, fear, anxiety)

Cognitive distancing

Denial

Proportioning (between catastrophizing and minimizing)

Omnipotent thinking (supercompetence)

Vigilant focusing (choosing a narrow, selective emphasis)

Search for spiritual meaning and hope

Tackling the illness (parents learning about the disease and implementing treatment regimen)

Showing the works (demonstrating insulin injections, sharing information with others)

Evidence of Coping

Acceptance of the illness

Adherence to the treatment regimen

Acknowledgment of challenges, responsibilities, limitations

Pursuit of age-appropriate peer and family relationships

Success with developmental tasks (e.g., academic performance)

Coping Resources and Moderators

Social support, especially family environment

Self-esteem

Ego development (defined as a "manifestation of integrative functioning involving impulse control, moral development, and quality of interpersonal relationships")

Health beliefs (regarding ability to influence their health)

Type A behavior (related to increased autonomic reactivity and blood glucose levels)

Temperament

Implications for Treatment

Each coping process, moderator, or resource may serve as a focus for intervention.

Matching a diabetes education program to level of ego development is likely to enhance effectiveness.

Intensive multicomponent care recipients show greater improvement than standard care recipients, although no one variable in the mix has been identified yet.

Approaches need to be family oriented, focused, and developmentally targeted.

Targets of Intervention

Adherence behavior

Knowledge of diabetes

Personality styles or traits amenable to change

Family processes such as support or conflict

The implications for treatment and targets of intervention summarized above combine psychological and educational facets that practitioners can weave into an effective psychotherapeutic approach to meet the goal set at the beginning of the chapter: to foster enough safety, security, regularity, and predictability of life for natural growth and healthy development to occur.

A comprehensive coping paradigm incorporates educational, developmental, cognitive, dynamic, interpersonal, systems, and social bases. These elements make it a sophisticated and heuristic conceptualization with wide application possibilities now and in the future. Despite the need and despite the good treatment possibilities, only a small proportion of chronically ill children receive the psychological assistance that could enhance their adaptation and development markedly. For example, Cadman, Boyle, Szatmari, and Offord (1987) reported that only 25% of children with chronic health problems and psychological disorders use mental health and social support services. Hymovich and Hagopian (1992) cited parents' use of support services as a major coping strategy, yet a discrepancy remains between the need for psychological services and the availability of community practitioners with adequate training in health-related clinical practice.

Case study: Emma and her horse. Emma was 8 years old when she and her parents discovered that she had type I diabetes. For the rest of her life, she would have to cope with daily injections, urine and blood tests, and dietary restrictions. At a time in life when initiative and the mastering of skills are in developmental focus, Emma became overwhelmed with things to do, most of which she did not want to do.

By the time Emma was 10 years old, she had been in the hospital three times with diabetic acidosis. On one of those occasions, she nearly died. Her parents worked hard to help her adjust to her disease. They tried special events, bribes, and even punishments at times, but Emma cried with every injection and ate cookies whenever she could sneak them. Her parents tried to tell her she was "special," but Emma felt only "strange." She avoided other children rather than let them know something was "wrong" with her.

Events were out of control when Emma's parents sought psychological help. Emma's father was a farmer with long work hours. Her mother was at home full-time, but she had five other children to care for, in addition to Emma. The mother was well-informed about diabetes, but she was discouraged because life with Emma involved a constant struggle for control. Neither the diabetes nor Emma seemed manageable.

In the course of talking with Emma and her family, the therapist learned that Emma's most fervent wish was to ride a horse. A plan was formed to allow riding lessons, in exchange for which she agreed to stop sneaking food. The therapist also taught Emma and her parents new distraction techniques for injection times. By the time Emma was 11 years old, she was a good rider. At that time, her parents decided to buy her a horse of her own and added a small stable to their farm.

At the psychologist's urging, Emma's mother encouraged Emma to learn to care for the horse. As Emma fed, watered, and groomed the animal that was five times her size, she began to feel competent at something for the first time. She was pleased when other children wanted to visit in order to learn to ride and help tend her horse. Emma began to feel "special."

The competence Emma developed in caring for her horse carried over into competence in caring for herself. With her psychologist's support and her mother's help, she mastered the skill of giving her own daily insulin injections. She was able to do her own "finger sticks" several times a day to check her blood sugar counts. By the time she was 12 years old, Emma was comfortable with these tasks and was socially comfortable with other children.

Emma's story encompasses a 4-year process, with periodic psychological intervention as needed, in which an overwhelmed diabetic child learned to cope with her disease and integrate its presence into her life. Emma was a latency age child whose need to develop mastery in the world beyond family, with school tasks and social relationships, was thwarted by the onset of a serious illness. Diabetic education alone was insufficient to address the turmoil in this particular child. She was not able to accept the illness or adhere to treatment as long as she felt different from and inferior to others. The therapist recommended that Emma attend a diabetic camp to facilitate sharing and self-esteem. The camp experience was growth enhancing for her. However, it was her affection for horses and a developing love for her own horse that provided the necessary emotional mainstay for Emma's adaptation. Through learning to ride and caring for the horse, she learned to meet challenges and responsibilities with growing skill. Riding gave her a much needed feeling of freedom, joy, and exhilaration as well.

Emma provides a good example of a child who needed intermittent, not continuous, psychological treatment. Over the 4-year period, she had no more than 30 psychotherapy sessions. The components of distraction techniques, camp (the group experience), and the unique tailoring of treatment to her special interest enabled her to move along a response continuum toward adaptation and growth.

Adolescence and the Developmental Hurdles

Adolescents are on the bridge between childhood and adulthood, sometimes seeming quite babylike and at other times seeming quite mature and self-possessed. The developmental tasks of the teen years are centered around making the transition to independent adulthood:

1. Adolescents must come to grips with adult sexuality—from the appearance of secondary sex characteristics at the beginning of adolescence to handling sexual impulses in themselves (and others who show sexual interest or rejection), to trial romantic relationships as they progress through adolescence.

2. They must loosen the dependent ties to parents—a process that has been called a *second individuation* by Blos (1967). Meeks (1986) believed it is more than a recapitulation of earlier development, because adolescents relate to others (parents and peers) primarily in a narcissistic mode, in response to the unpredictability of body changes, the upsurge of sexual and aggressive impulses, and the need to devalue parents.

3. They must develop autonomy and a coherent sense of identity—paradoxically sought throughout adolescence in the focus on their peers for support and mirroring of their efforts to both belong and break away simultaneously. The search for individuation and autonomy includes forays into the world of work, as young adult contributors to society.

Adolescents with a chronic illness and their parents must manage these major tasks even while the exigencies of the illness may exert a strong pull away from sexuality, dating, separation, autonomy, social time with peers, education or vocational preparation, and the overall goal of independence. Adolescence is an unstable phase of life under normal circumstances, with identity formation proceeding with the starts and bumps and stops of experimentation. It comes as no surprise to most clinicians that the volatility of mood and behavior associated with the adolescent stage of development affects the teen's handling of the illness and vice versa.

Treatment Issues

Treatment for the adolescent can be tailored to support their need for dual goals:

- Goal 1: To identify and enhance areas of autonomy and independence over their bodily functions, their need for a peer social network, their need to experiment and foster identity development.
- Goal 2: To accept the necessary dependence on medical treatment regimens and on other people for assistance with physical needs.

Problems develop when adolescents find themselves unable to move toward both goals. Body image, desirability, and fertility are affected by drugs, surgeries, and disabilities. Adolescents and their parents may be reluctant to discuss these areas related to sexuality directly or may deny the impact altogether, at least for a time. One oncological gynecologist informed us that often she must tell adolescent girls who have been previously treated for cancer and their mothers that the result of those treatments is ovarian failure and infertility. Although they had been told at the time of cancer treatment of the hormonal consequences, most of them still hoped it would not be true for them. Hearing the news again brings on distress and sadness as they face the loss. Another gynecological problem faced by adolescent girls who have been immunosuppressed by disease and treatments is their very high susceptibility to infections (genital warts, herpes, candidiasis) once they become sexually active. These girls can reduce the likelihood of infection with the use of condoms, if they can be helped to acknowledge both their sexual activity and their need to protect themselves physically.

Adolescent boys seem less concerned, in general, with fertility, and more concerned with prowess. The dominant worry of one 17-year-old male patient was loss of status in the eyes of the other male teenagers in his school group after he developed diabetes. Once a popular athlete, proud of his body, he became ashamed of the body he felt had betrayed him at the rising height of his physical strength. If he could not attract girls and play sports, how could he feel manly around the other teens? Another male patient, just entering adolescence, had many body concerns, and fertility was among them. He had been treated for juvenile rheumatoid arthritis since the age of 4 with large doses of steroids. Each time his physician tried to wean the steroids out of his body, the painful joint swelling flared again and the steroids were resumed. The disease and the steroid treatment resulted in his stunted growth, reduced and hampered participation in soccer (his favorite sport), and a permanently damaged right wrist that made writing and fine motor tasks difficult. At the age of 13, he made an appointment with the family physician he had known for most of his life. He arrived with a notebook containing questions about his future. He wanted to know if he would continue to grow and how tall he would get. He wanted to know if his condition would improve enough to play soccer on a team. He wanted to know if he could marry. The physician thought the last question reflected his worry about girls finding him attractive, but he clarified that his concern was based on whether he would ever be able to have children. The physician was surprised at his maturity. It was not possible at the time to ascertain whether the immunosuppressants had compromised his fertility. Most children grow out of juvenile rheumatoid arthritis; that is, the disease flare-ups stop. Few people realize, as this teen did, that the residual damage caused by the disease and its treatment persists throughout life.

Power struggles may erupt with parents or the medical team, the outward sign of an internal battle between the need for both independence and dependence. Often, an adolescent correctly assesses his or her ability to handle a situation satisfactorily, but one or both parents take an overprotective stance out of anxiety and concern for their child's safety. In this situation, the parents unwittingly thwart moves toward attainable levels of independence. At other times, the same adolescent may show poor judgment about capacities or consequences because of a strong desire to act on an impulse, or fit into a peer group, or run away from the illness. It is a very difficult parenting job to set limits under these circumstances. Taking a family systems perspective, McDaniel, Hepworth, and Doherty (1992) have pointed out the painful position of parents who are held responsible for the child's compliance by the medical team when they are without the wherewithal to ensure that compliance. The struggling adolescent's drama can pit parents against each other, family members and the medical team against each other, and the adolescent against any or all adults or siblings.

Psychological treatment strategies associated with illness must be responsive to the adolescent's place on the developmental spectrum. For example, Levenson et al. (1982) identified information preferences for 11- to 20-year-old cancer patients, as follows: 68% of patients preferred private discussions, particularly with physicians; 68% would include parents in the discussions; however, those under 15 years of age were most likely to prefer information from parents only. We see in this study the developmental shift typical of the stage of life.

Case Study

Mary Agnes was a 17-year-old with cystic fibrosis when she entered psychological treatment because of her distress in dealing with her parents. At the suggestion of the psychologist, her parents agreed to enter treatment also, construing their participation as a means to help their daughter. The focal conflict in the family centered on a dispute over autonomy. Mary Agnes wanted more freedom—to go away to college, to embark on the career she had chosen (pediatric nursing) as the most meaningful contribution she could make. She emphasized how important the nursing care she received throughout her childhood had been to her own sense of comfort and hope. She also wanted to be a giver of care, rather than always a receiver of care. Mary Agnes's parents, however, were understandably anxious about her plans and her pulling away from them. They were afraid for her life if she were to encounter a respiratory crisis and they were not available to assist her. They were afraid she would feel defeated and stigmatized if she were to be rejected by all the programs because of her health status. They were afraid of facing the loss brought on by separation, because each year she survived and thrived seemed too precious to relinquish any time with her.

The treatment focus centered on integration of the polarizing split between Mary Agnes and her parents, enabling her to move forward toward life-enhancing goals. With the help of the psychologist (and consultation with her medical team), she was able to establish her program of necessary self-care, equipment needs, and emergency procedures and to select only schools that could provide access to medical care continuity. Then she was able to assuage her parents' realistic concerns about her safety. With help, her parents were able to join with and take pleasure in her aspirations, while coming to terms with their own loss inherent in their daughter's growing up. The resolution was appropriate for the developmental phase of late adolescence and appropriate for her enduring personal needs, which are shaped by the impact of cystic fibrosis. Mary Agnes, now a 23-year-old nurse, works with children on a pediatric unit in a community hospital.

Summary

Not all children and adolescents who have chronic illnesses will have problems with adaptation, but illness precipitates a strain on them that has major repercussions for their physical, psychological, and social growth and development. All children with illness and disability are at increased risk for a decrement in psychological function. The psychologically healthiest youngsters grow to experience themselves fully and are not limited to an identity based primarily on the disease. They grow into adults who can work and love, who can give and take, who can balance independence and dependence. The most psychologically vulnerable youngsters and families, who show poorer adjustment patterns, can be helped with psychotherapeutic approaches based on trauma resolution and coping enhancement that are sensitive to changing developmental needs over the life span.

Chapter 9

The Family and Chronic Illness

An individual with chronic illness is not an isolated entity. "A person has the illness and that illness is embedded within a network of people who also are affected by the illness. Their families interact with larger societal organizations to assist and cope with illness in one of their members" (McDaniel et al., 1992, p. 16).

For years, illness was seen only as a function of the disease and the individual patient. In the late 1970s, George Engel proposed a "biopsychosocial model" for illness that included not only the patient and the disease, but also the larger hierarchy of individuals and groups to which the patient belonged. In 1980, he elaborated on this in an article he published in the *American Journal of Psychiatry* (see Figure 1).

Chronic illness affects the patient profoundly, and an understanding of the disease, the individual's intrapsychic premorbid personality structure, and the response of the patient who struggles to adapt to physical illness is essential to psychological treatment. In this chapter, patients are discussed in the context of their near and extended families. First, interpersonal support systems are considered in relation to the patient with chronic physical illness. Second, the family is examined as a provider of support. The third area of concern is the family as it is affected by the patient's illness. Last, the treatment of significant partners and family members is discussed. The goal of family treatment

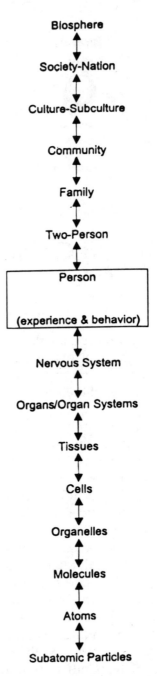

Figure 1. Systems hierarchy. From "The Clinical Application of the Biosocial Model," by G. L. Engel, 1980, *American Journal of Psychiatry, 137*, p. 537. Copyright 1980 by the American Psychiatric Association. Reprinted by permission.

is to enable a family to provide better support for the patient's needs and manage the impact of the illness on individual family members and the family system as a whole.

Many psychotherapists are not trained to work with families, and it may not always be in the individual patient's best interest for the same therapist to work with both the patient and the family members. The goal of this discussion is to explain to psychotherapists the needs and problems that arise in the context of the family and to suggest referral and coordinate psychotherapy of family members and the family unit when necessary.

Interpersonal Support Systems

Social support influences the way in which an individual adapts to illness (Koocher & O'Malley, 1981; Morrow et al., 1981). In some cases, social support also seems to influence the actual outcomes of illness (Funch & Marshall, 1983; Weisman & Worden, 1975). Broadhead et al. (1983), in an extensive epidemiological review of the literature on social support, concluded that

> social support is much more than a simple environmental exposure. It can be studied as an effect modifier or buffer against the stress of life events, but also as a direct determinant of health or illness (an independent variable) and as dependent variable with its own causes and determinants. (p. 533)

It is not clear exactly how social support works or how the effectiveness of social support can be measured. Rowland (1989) prepared five criteria for the assessment of social support: the type of support, the source of support (providers), the quantity and availability of support, the quality and content of support given, and the perceived need for support.

Types of Supports

Emotional–affectional support may be the most helpful type of support, but other types of support are also important. For example, tangible support (financial and physical help) for an unemployed young adult suffering from chronic fatigue syndrome may be more helpful than any other form of assistance. Educational support may be invaluable and actually prolong the lives of patients with diabetes or asthma. Affirmational support to cancer patients who have finished medical treatment and are about to be on their own can enable them to begin to resume their former lives. Without a sense of being understood and supported, they might instead feel isolated and withdraw from life further than their disease would mandate. Without a sense of belonging— affiliational support from family and friends—patients can become further isolated and become physically ill again if they retreat into illness. The type of support needed depends on the disease itself, the phase of the disease process (acute, chronic, or resolving), and the individual.

An interesting model by Schulz and Rau (1985) provides a view of life course events in terms of their statistical and temporal normality. For example, terminal illness at age 75 is accepted as normal. The onset of a chronic illness beginning at age 3 years, such as diabetes, is not normal for a child, the parents, siblings, or extended family. The types of support needed in the latter situation are different from those needed in the case of the elderly person whose life expectancy is nearly complete.

It is important to be aware of the type of support needed. It can be completely unsupportive to explore past childhood conflicts when one must instead think about managing illness. However, problems in managing the present needs sometimes reflect old, unresolved conflicts. Therefore, it can be unsupportive to focus entirely on the illness and to make an amalgam of the patient and the illness, because such a focus ignores the concerns and struggles that existed long before the onset of the chronic illness. A person's identity is larger than his or her role as a patient. Perhaps the best way to evaluate the type of support needed is to find sufficient congruence between the adaptive requirements of a task and the type of support.

Source of Support

Who is the source of support? Most often it is a family member, but not always. One of the important tasks in assessing social support is to identify the source of support. One way to discover the sources of support is to think in terms of tasks that need to be done, as the contributors to *Breast Cancer: A Psychological Treatment Manual* (Haber, 1995) have done. Who provides emotional support, or who listens to the patient? Who helps with treatment decisions? Who helps with caretaking demands? Who helps with ongoing family demands? All of these questions represent various needs of the chronically ill person.

Often, parents take care of ill children; spouses or significant others take care of their partners. But when a caregiver must work and maintain a career to provide income, for example, then who steps in? In one family, the wife was severely debilitated by diabetes and the complications of medication therapy. For several months, her husband was able to take time away from his job as a state employee. When his leave was over and his wife still needed daily home care and transportation to rehabilitation and physician facilities, both his and her elderly parents attempted to fill the need, but the demands were too great for these aging parents. Finally, after a difficult search, community resources were found and enlisted, which provided relief for the strained family system.

Quantity and Availability of Support

The quantity and availability of support may be best evaluated by examining the patients' family system, membership in social and professional groups, and social contacts.

For example, the diabetic disabled woman in the previous example had a spouse who was able and willing to support her as long as he could stay home. He continued to provide emotional support after he returned to work. The couple's elderly parents attempted to meet caretaking demands, but their availability was markedly limited by their own infirmities and their distance from the patient's home.

An exploration of the couple's pre-illness social structure revealed that, like many Northeasterners, they lived in one state and worked in another. The very specialized treatment needed by the wife could not be provided locally. When she was at home, her caretaking needs necessitated support from nearby friends and neighbors. One of the most difficult management tasks facing this woman was finding help to make long trips to the large city medical center, at least once or twice a week at times of medical crises. Eventually, help was obtained from a group of neighbors who rotated trips into the city.

Quality of Support

Assessing the quality of support is difficult. In the previous example, the couple described almost any help as "wonderful," whereas the patient's mother described the quality of support as "meager" and "inadequate." The mother felt this strongly, because she was the person most often called for backup support when rides or home help fell through. She would go frequently to help her daughter on short notice, even though she lived 1-1/2 hours away from the patient, had arthritis, and had to deal with her husband's chronic disability with Parkinson's disease. To assess the quality of support, it is important to solicit information periodically not only from the person receiving support, but also from the person rendering support.

Perceived Need for Support

In assessing support, one must also examine the perceived need of the patient. In the case presented above, the young woman who perceived her support as "wonderful" did so because she was ashamed of her neediness and was unwilling to be a "burden" on anyone. She labeled all support as "more than she wanted," but she had difficulty acknowledging how much help she really needed. Eventually, with considerable psychotherapy, she was able to acknowledge her need for support and was able to establish more dependable systems than those she had arranged early in her illness.

Attempts to provide unwanted support are ultimately doomed to failure. Either providing support or receiving support may be difficult when dealing with the problems of chronic physical illness. Many people are comfortable giving support in a short-term situation but cannot provide support through the long duration of chronic illness. Other people respond to crises poorly but can provide support quietly and consistently for long periods. Most people react to illness by wishing it would go away and by hoping it will not affect them personally. These attitudes, which are discussed in the countertransference chapter, also affect support givers and families.

The Family as a Support System

Who Is the Family?

The term *family* includes all people who have kin relationships or are significant others and have "kinlike" relationships. The term *significant other* refers to heterosexual individuals who live together intimately but are not formally acknowledged as kin. It also refers to homosexual couples who are partners and share an intimate relationship over time. Special problems arise from these less formal relationships, which were introduced in chapter 7. Family members involved with patients may be members of the immediate family who live together, grandparents, children who have left home, aunts, uncles, and cousins.

In the example of the debilitated chronically ill diabetic woman referred to earlier, the family included her spouse and both his and her parents. The couple, in their late 30s, had no children. Each had one sibling who lived more than 1,000 miles away. Although each sibling was too far away to be able to form part of the support network for the patient, each sibling was affected by the demands of the illness. One sibling in particular felt cheated of his parents' time.

In some families the family unit consists only of siblings. One group of elderly sisters lived together harmoniously until one of them became chronically ill. Two of the women had been married and widowed; the third sister had never married. One of the widowed sisters had had children who had died; the other had none. When the eldest unmarried sister became severely handicapped by arthritis, the others had to pitch in and physically wash and dress her. The task was easier for the two widowed siblings to do than it was for the patient herself to accept. The patient's discomfort caused significant family disruption.

Spouses are the most frequent source of support. As is often the case, however, the spouse can be unavailable because he or she earns the family income. This was the case in the family of the diabetic woman. With elderly couples, spouses may be physically present but so infirm that they cannot provide either emotional or caretaking support. When one partner is deteriorating from a disease such as Alzheimer's or Parkinson's, the well spouse may pull away and be unwilling to provide support of any kind. The well spouse sees no hope of any future relationship with the deteriorating partner.

Parents are the next most common supporters of patients with chronic illness. In the case of young children with cancer, asthma, or diabetes, one person (usually the mother) provides direct physical care and one provides financial care. The parents in turn can (one hopes) support each other emotionally. The popular film Lorenzo's Oil gives a very poignant picture of the way in which parents may struggle to meet the needs of a chronically ill, debilitated child. It shows, too, their attempts to nurture each other throughout a long illness. In single-parent families, the struggle to provide both physical and financial care can become overwhelming.

At times, children become the principal support providers in a family system. Even young children may be the primary providers of support for ill parents. Adult children with aging, ill parents frequently provide emotional, physical, and financial support. Alice bravely supported her husband through a year and a half of painful prostate cancer. Shortly after his death she was diagnosed with colon cancer. She became debilitated rapidly and needed either intensive home care or nursing home placement. At first, the adult children felt unable to provide care for their mother because they were overwhelmed by their father's recent painful death. With supportive psychotherapy, however, the children were able to grieve and then to provide round-the-clock care of their mother. She eventually died at home, in the presence of all three children. All the children in this family sought psychotherapy following their mother's death. All were glad they had been able to take care of their mother, despite the associated difficulties.

Ability to Adapt to Chronic Illness

Not all families can adapt to chronic physical illness. Several variables affect the family's ability to adapt. In general, the family's history of flexibility in stressful situations can predict the ability to adapt to the chronic illness of a particular member. One elderly woman had a malignant breast mass. Her husband, nieces, and friends all gathered around as she made decisions for mastectomy and aftercare. She and her spouse had a long history of talking about problems and working them out together, with help from church friends and extended family.

Another patient of the same age refused to tell her husband or daughter about her uterine cancer, discovered on biopsy in the physician's office. She refused treatment repeatedly. Concerned, the doctor called in the husband and, eventually, the daughter. Communication was neither usual nor easy for this family. After many delays, she agreed to treatment, and her recovery from surgery was prolonged. Eventually, the spouse began to accompany the woman on her visits to the physician. The patient's daughter was educated about the mother's need for regular checkups and provided transportation. This family did not communicate well with each other. Under stress, family members tended to separate from each other, making it hard for the family to be supportive of the patient in any way. It is important to assess the family's way of dealing with stress, its flexibility, and the ability of the various members to communicate.

Phase of the Illness

A family's ability to adapt to chronic illness also varies with the phase of illness. Many families can organize and coordinate support for an ill member in the acute phase of an illness. Gerald, a 58-year-old man, had a heart attack while at work, where he was the head of the company. His wife and three children supported him emotionally and concretely through his illness and rehabilitation. However, he was severely incapacitated by his illness and had to sell his business.

Gerald's wife resumed her work, which was necessary to enable the family to maintain its lifestyle. As time passed and Gerald entered the chronic phase of illness, he needed less intensive care. He could do some things for himself but had to wait for other things until his wife got home from work or his children from school. An authoritarian man, accustomed to his role as head of the household, Gerald would insist that people be at specific places at certain times. At the beginning of the chronic phase of illness, the family mustered forces and provided the support he demanded, because they were used to pulling together under his direction. As the chronic phase of the illness progressed and family members struggled to make a living and live their own lives, they found it more and more difficult to respond to the father's dictatorial style. Gerald was unwilling to consult a psychotherapist, but his wife did. The children left home, one of them quite prematurely. Eventually, the wife left her spouse to his own devices. The entire family came apart, unable to support their ill member or to restructure themselves as a family unit. They had worked together with remarkable cooperation at the onset of illness but were unable to tolerate the chronic phase. They were too inflexible to adjust their roles and ways of communicating with each other.

On the other hand, some families tolerate chronic illness but come apart in the resolution phase of illness, particularly when the resolution is death. Individuals may tolerate chronicity because relationships, while altered, still exist. As death approaches, however, fears of abandonment may arise, or there may be guilt about survival. Some family members may withdraw support at this time to seek other relationships and support for themselves. Still other families can unite during the termination phase of an illness, because they perceive an end of the chaos in their lives caused by the chronic illness. In one such family, the patriarch of nine children was dying of liver cancer. He had been ill for 2 years prior to his last hospitalization. His two ex-wives and nine children had not spoken to each other for several months. The patient adamantly refused to speak to a daughter who had chosen to have a child out of wedlock. As he and family members began to realize he was dying, they began to talk to one another, to forgive one another. Over a period of several weeks, the new grandchild of the ostracized daughter was brought to the hospital at the request of the patient. In the end, the family were with the patient constantly and were speaking among themselves in ways they had not in many years. The entire family, including both ex-wives, were at his bedside when he died.

Family Life Cycle

Another important variable in a family's ability to adapt to chronic illness and provide support is the family's place in its life cycle.

Rolland (1987) has written extensively on the interface between illness and the family and individual life cycle. Combrinck-Graham (1985) has described a family life spiral, which is shown graphically in Figure 2. She described a person's and family's reciprocal relationships with each other at different stages of life. At times of childbearing, for example, the family focuses on taking care of its members. In late adolescence and early adulthood, the focus of individuals is on separating from one another and establishing independence.

Joe and Mary had been married 3 years when Joe's father developed Alzheimer's disease. His mother had a long history of diabetes, which was controlled with diet. At the time of the Alzheimer's diagnosis, Mary and Joe had just had their first child after a long struggle with fertility problems. They had supported each other throughout the infertility workup, and now a complicated delivery had left Mary physically drained and in need of help. Joe needed to spend more time with his parents at a time when his wife needed more support in caring for their newborn. Joe's mother responded to the increased stress in trying to care for her husband and maintain her job by eating, which made her diabetes worse. At the same time, she did not want to draw Joe away from his family; she wanted to support her children and develop her role as grandmother to her long-awaited grandchild.

A powerful force pulled Joe from his new family back into his family of origin. He wanted to help his mother cope with his father's Alzheimer's disease and protect her from worsening diabetes, but it was an impossible task. Gradually, Joe and his mother, with support in two cities from two family therapists and two physicians, placed the father in a home for Alzheimer's patients. As they relaxed and realized he was comfortable, Joe and his mother were able to resume the normal cycle of their

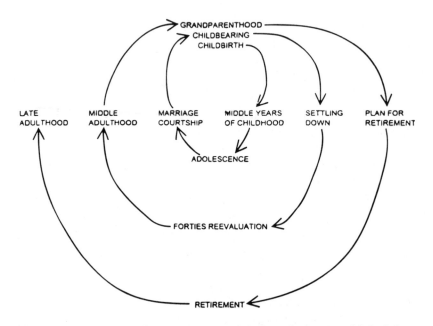

Figure 2. Family life spiral. From "A Developmental Model for Family Systems," by L. Combrinck-Graham, 1985, *Family Process*, 24, p. 142. Copyright 1985 by Family Process, Inc. Reprinted with permission.

lives. Joe enjoyed becoming an active parent, and Joe's mother became a helpful, supportive grandmother. They all visited Joe's father regularly; he no longer recognized them, but laughed with them at the baby's antics, enjoying her in his way.

Compare Joe's family with Rita's. Rita and Rich had three children. Rita was at home taking care of her young family when her mother became ill with breast cancer. Because Rita was at home full-time with small children, she was able to take the children with her readily to visit her mother and run errands for her. Prior to illness, they were in the habit of visiting Rita's family on weekends. Caring for her mother was indeed an added burden for Rita, but it did not significantly pull her away from her family. The family relationships were close between children, parents, and grandparents at the time of the grandmother's illness. Thus, adapting to illness was less stressful for Rita and her family than for Joe and his new family.

The comparison continues with a third family. Deidre was graduating from college at the time her mother developed ovarian cancer. She turned down the marketing job she had accepted before her mother's diagnosis and returned home to care for her mother so that her father could continue his work and her younger brother could leave for college. The job of caring for her mother extended into Deidre's late 20s, affecting her career and marriage plans. At the very time in life when she should have been going off on her own, she was needed at home to provide support to her mother.

The family's ability to adapt to a member with chronic illness depends on its ability to adapt to stress. This ability varies with the stage of illness (acute, chronic, or resolution) and with the family's place in its life cycle at the time illness occurs.

Effects of Chronic Illness on the Family

Although the family can be a provider of support, some of the above examples demonstrate that the family itself is profoundly affected by a member's chronic illness and may need support. Some families can adapt. Some, like Gerald's family, completely disintegrate. Some individuals, like Deidre, are so deeply affected that they have difficulty restructuring the lives that were completely altered by a family member's illness. Families of chronically ill patients should be evaluated early in the treatment process. Support and intervention may prevent the breakdown of the family or its individual members. The therapist should be aware of a patient's support system, the involvement of the patient's family in that support system, the effect of the patient's illness on the family, and the life cycle of the family.

Therapists should also consider a family's structure. The family is a complex unit of subsystems in which individuals relate to each other along hierarchical lines. Some of these systems are inflexible, as was the case with Gerald's family. Other systems, although highly organized, can be redefined, as in the family of three elderly siblings. In order to adapt as a unit with the patient's arthritis, each of the three sisters had to arrange new boundaries. Receiving physical care from a sibling and giving physical care to a sibling created new roles for each member of the family. Roles and boundaries had to change in this family.

Therapists must gather information about the family's history and beliefs about illness. For example, when illness has occurred in the past, how did the family respond and what are the beliefs about illness? David had colon cancer. He was adamant about refusing treatment. He had long conversations with his physician regarding his refusal to have a relatively simple, potentially life-saving surgery. In the course of inquiring about illness in other family members, the physician learned that the patient's maternal uncle had died of colon cancer. David, along with his mother and her family, believed the uncle died because the surgery spread the disease by seeding it throughout his body. The family belief about illness explained the patient's refusal to get the help he needed. Once this belief was uncovered and corrected, he began to be more flexible about getting proper medical treatment.

Another area of resistance concerned the family–treatment interface. David seemed to understand and accept the information provided by his physician, which clarified and educated him about his uncle's operation and death. In fact, he had obtained records of his uncle's surgery and gone over the differences between his uncle's stage of disease and his own. Yet he kept deferring surgery. Why?

Although David had been educated, his wife and mother had not. They still held the family belief about illness and regularly pleaded with him not to have the surgery. Treatment did not proceed until the whole family was brought in for several sessions with the physician, to discuss their beliefs and receive accurate information about this disease. David's family was very involved in decisions about his treatment. When this was understood and they became part of the treatment team, definitive treatment could proceed.

Treatment of the Family

Ideally, when a person has a chronic physical illness, an assessment of the family should include gathering information about the disease and the ordeal the family will be up against; the point in the family life cycle at which the disease occurs; the family structure; the family history and beliefs about illness; and the ways in which a family relates to the treatment setting. This assessment should enable the therapist to anticipate problems and enable the individual and the family to adapt effectively to chronic illness. Perhaps someday such a goal will be attainable. In reality, early assessment of the family rarely happens. According to Rait and Lederberg (1990), families come into therapy under three different circumstances: first, when they fail in supportive care of the member with chronic illness; second, when an individual member has an obvious psychiatric need; third, when friction between patient, staff, and family is severe enough to interfere with the patient's treatment needs. The therapist who is working with a chronically ill patient should think about the patient's family as early in the process as possible. Inquiring about support and the family structure is useful so that help can be provided to the family before a crisis occurs.

The broad goals of family treatment are rather straightforward: to provide support and to enable the family to restructure itself in order to cope with the demand of chronic illness. Support for the family and its members can be thought of in much the same terms described previously in this chapter—in terms of support type, source, quantity and availability, quality, and perceived need.

When family members come for help, they most often need emotional and educational support. Listening to family members and enabling them to express their unacceptable thoughts about the patient and the illness are two of the most supportive things the therapist can do. Simply being able to express such utterances as "I wish he were dead," or "I can't stand to bathe my sister" can provide great relief for the individual who is burdened with guilt and afraid expression of such thought may worsen the illness. These ideas are common among people who must care for chronically ill family members. Affects such as anger, anxiety, and grief are often overwhelming to family members as well as patients. Again, listening and facilitating expression of disturbing feelings can be immensely helpful.

Educational support is often needed to understand the disease process and the ordeal the family must prepare to endure. One can refer the family to the physician or to support groups relating to a particular illness. Family group meetings with the collaborating therapist and physician are among the most helpful forms of education. Therapists may function as advocates to help families question and clarify how the disease will affect them. In such meetings it is often possible to identify what types of support the individual and family will need and who will provide it. In addition to educating families, these joint meetings can help the health care provider understand the limits of the family system in providing support, as well as the resources available within the family.

Family therapy should help a family identify external support systems such as churches, schools, and support groups specific to the illness, and it should enable members to learn how to gain access to such support. It is also helpful and necessary to understand what support a family thinks it needs. Needs will vary according to the family's sense of itself. Some families need to keep to themselves and provide as much of their own support as possible. This strategy can work, depending on the demands of the illness, the duration of the illness, the life stage of the family, and other family resources. It can be frustrating, fruitless work to attempt to impose outside systems of support on the family that does not want them. Other families are unwilling or unable to provide support for their ill member and themselves and feel safe only when they are attached to multiple outside systems of support. Good supportive therapy after careful assessment enables the family to make as good a match as possible between its perceived needs and available resources.

In addition to providing support, therapy for the family of the chronically ill patient should enable the family to restructure itself to cope with the demands of the illness and the ill patient. Depending on the pre-illness structure of the family and the nature of the disease, as well as the stage of the life cycle, some families will require more facilitative help than others. All families will experience some degree of disorganization in response to chronic illness. The objectives of the restructuring of the family are to provide a family system that incorporates but is not structured solely around the illness; to provide a system that facilitates the developmental tasks of all members; and to provide a system that is able to nurture and support not only the chronically ill patient, but also each member of the group.

One of the ways in which restructuring the family can be facilitated is to improve communication among family members. This can be done in the therapist's office with the whole family present. There are also community groups in which several different families gather together and share their feelings. Some groups are restricted to siblings or spouses. The family group environment often facilitates communication in a safe, permissible way between family members.

Another important way of facilitating family restructuring is to respect the defenses of individual members. A family member who feels unable to care for a patient with bed sores can often be a good provider of concrete financial and emotional support. Arranging for outside help respects the individual's defenses. It enables family members to give what they are able to give.

Facilitating a family's sense of agency, its ability to act on its own behalf, in the face of overwhelming illness is yet another strategy to help restructure a family. In the case of Alice, her children felt overwhelmed by the loss of their father and by the imminent loss of their mother. Helping these adult children grieve for their father enabled them to be able to act on their wish to care for their mother in the terminal phase of her illness. Continued work with the sadness and anger generated by their mother's illness facilitated a sense of increased ability to cope with the profound illness in the family. In the final phase of illness, they felt pleased with what they had accomplished. Each of these children experienced themselves and their family as stronger and more capable than before the mother's illness. The grief work facilitated this family's sense of agency. It helped them emerge from their ordeal as a restructured unit that was able to nurture and support both the chronically ill member and themselves.

In summary, the family is one of an individual's primary resources for help in dealing with chronic illness. The family, in turn, is deeply affected by the individual member's protracted illness. Adequate psychotherapy for the patient with chronic physical illness will consider the family both as an available resource and as a unit affected by the illness. Treatment will involve support for the individual patient as well as arranging for or providing support and restructuring for the family of the patient with chronic illness.

10

A Case Summary: The Psychological Treatment of a Kidney Transplant Patient

Solange* was a young woman who entered psychotherapy with symptoms of depression following major life change: serious illness, major surgery (a kidney transplant), and the necessity for lifelong adjustments to the consequences of chronic disease. As a summary of the holographic model of illness, we discuss Solange from the multiple views, angles, and dimensions presented throughout the text. Then we present the narrative case treatment summary of Solange in a format familiar to most practitioners. Certainly, many other kinds of approaches and interventions would have been possible. Each therapist must work within his or her knowledge base and make the best choices possible within the confines of his or her own experience, personality, and setting.

The Templates

The disease templates provide an explanation of the nature of Solange's illness. The Medical Template categorizes disease by outcome, process, etiology, and needs. Solange developed thrombocytopenic purpura, which soon led to renal failure and

---

*Not her real name. Some demographic and other details have been omitted in order to protect her privacy.

dialysis (outcome and process). Treatment with a transplanted kidney led to a lifelong requirement for immunosuppressive medication (management needs). The etiology of the illness was not clear, but the disease was very similar to that of Solange's mother and may have a genetic component. Solange's management needs included thinking about future life events such as pregnancy, an option that could be life threatening at worst and difficult at best. Other management needs involved dietary restrictions and her increased need for rest.

In terms of the Threat Template, Solange's present disease is understood (a transplanted kidney) and manageable (medication). However, her kidney could fail, as did her friend's just prior to her entrance into psychotherapy. If the kidney fails, the disease could become life threatening again and very difficult to manage.

The Response Template is represented by Solange's search for help. Solange came for psychological help very late in her disease progression, when overwhelmed by grief. Her disease onset was abrupt, severe, and debilitating. She could not expend internal resources during the phase of acute illness to process the experience; that was possible only after her health was stabilized and her condition reached chronic manageable proportions. She had cycled rapidly through the sequence of recognizing something was wrong, continued to be wrong, and was disturbing her life.

The decision to risk transplant surgery, with the hope of preserving her life, was the response to a desperate wish for a cure. This part of the response cycle is impelled by the idea that whatever is wrong has to be changed. In her case it was an appropriate choice and was recommended by her medical team. The dramatic improvement in her body with a new and functioning kidney cannot be overestimated. Her life improved as well. Over time, she began to assimilate what had happened to her and to recognize the chronic nature of the changes in her body. She started to recognize that she could not change what was wrong. She entered psychotherapy at the point in her responsiveness when she did not know how she could live with what was wrong and had changed her life. Psychotherapy helped her to grapple with the disorganizing experience and to begin to reconsolidate and adapt.

Solange's premorbid personality style and level of functioning (the Psychological Template) pointed toward a favorable prognosis for reconsolidation and adaptation. She was intelligent and had many internal and external resources. Managing reality did not present a problem for her. Her cognitive style of management was well organized and quietly thoughtful. She showed good judgment and problem-solving skills. On a fundamental level her relationship skills were mature, fluid, and easy. She was accustomed to give and take with her siblings and peers, knew how to share, got along well with others, and was comfortable with both men and women. On a deeper level, however, she had a self-protective and a protecting stance with authority figures, more with men than women. Therefore, she had a valence toward pleasing others and not asking for too much, lest she be criticized and risk losing needed support and attention. One would expect to see this valence carry over into an intimate relationship with a man and to be heightened during times of interpersonal conflict or when she had a greater need for support. Telltale signs of her self-protective ambivalent stance were already evident in her relationship with a specific man.

Anxiety was managed and held at bay with her beliefs about the need for self-discipline. She was able also to reach out to others and to be comforted by them. Her religious faith was an additional source of reassurance. She was overloaded when she arrived for psychotherapy, and her defenses, although quite functional, were failing her. Her feelings of helplessness, disorganization, and grief were normal reactions to the trauma endured; in fact, she was able to stave off the downward slide longer than most people could have done, thanks to the strength of her defenses against annihilation anxiety and loss. All in all, she had a significant capacity to bear feelings without complaint or uncontrollable anxiety.

Solange's mastery–competence level was high. Probably most of the patients in a general psychotherapy practice do not function quite so well at baseline. The interferences in her psychological capacity to move naturally into a productive and related adult life were not a function of a personality disorder. The interferences were a function of her disease process and the profound threat to her life.

The formative early life experience of death, with the loss of her mother and her father's subsequent inability to help her mourn, contributed a depressive cast to her personality. That did not constitute a diagnosis of major depression, but rather a recognition of the theme of loss, which could only be deepened by her illness. The need to mourn is a significant part of Solange's emotional landscape and structure.

Short-Term Dynamic Psychotherapy

The psychological treatment focused on the interwoven past and present themes of loss in an attempt to help Solange face her disorganization and gain stability. Consistent with the continuum of disorganization–reorganization–reconsolidation (described in chapter 5 with the specific associated themes in illness), three themes were addressed: body image changes associated with decreased self-esteem; mourning associated with loss; and negative affects associated with physical, psychological, and social discomfort.

From among the long menu of possible interventions, the primary approach chosen was a dynamically focused psychotherapy, which had to be carried out within a mandated, externally dictated, time-limited context. Some cognitive–behavioral components were integrated, such as the assignment of out-of-session tasks.

The choice of a short-term dynamic psychotherapy (STDP) carries with it some quite specific selection criteria and treatment methods if it is to benefit patients. Furthermore, the model must be modified for patients who have special difficulties because of their illness. STDP differs from long-term treatment in several ways. In STDP, the therapist is more active, especially in formulating and maintaining the focus. The technique limits the patient's dependence on the therapist and his or her regression, which tends to prevent the development of a transference neurosis. Transference valences, however, are always present. The working through phase is foreshortened, because the treatment ends before it can be completed. Despite their differences, both long- and short-term treatments are designed to result in improved adaptation.

For the best prognosis, patients should meet the following STDP criteria:

- have a clear problem focus,
- be able to form a relationship and to withstand separation,
- have ego-dystonic symptoms (i.e., the patient recognizes the problem as personally troublesome),
- be motivated to make use of help,
- have the capacity for introspection (psychological mindedness).

These criteria have been synthesized from among widely agreed on variables (see Flegenheimer, 1982; Goodheart, 1989; Malan, 1976; Mann, 1973; Messer & Warren, 1995; Strupp & Binder, 1984). Solange met the criteria. The requisite psychotherapy techniques are oriented toward initial, middle, and termination phases. The initial phase includes two main tasks, the establishment of a working therapeutic alliance and arrival at a mutually understood focus of concern. The middle phase is oriented toward an exploration and greater understanding of the patient's problems and the mobilization of his or her potential for change. In the termination phase, technique is centered around understanding the meaning of separation for the patient and managing the transition.

Goodheart (1989) explored modifications in STDP for difficult patients with special needs. Along with the more customary categories of patients with personality disorders, she included patients with physical loss, illness, or disability, as well as patients whose parents are psychologically dysfunctional (e.g., they have psychosis or addictions or are undifferentiated). In psychotherapy for ill patients,

> the struggles around body integrity become intertwined with character style. Examples of patients with physical problems who have been treated within a modified STDP model are those with mastectomy, kidney transplant, Turner's syndrome, infertility, and severe dyslexia. In many rehabilitation settings, counselors and medical workers do a fine job of helping people adapt to loss and limitation. However, these people often present themselves later for

treatment in other settings. At that point, it is not sufficient to work with just a body focus. The challenge to the clinician is to work with the tangled psyche-soma interactions, combined with the developmental phase of life and underlying personality structure. The difficulty for the patients is their need for reintegration, a process that cannot be hurried, but perhaps can be aided. (p. 18)

In general, the modifications were developed within a framework to allow working with the deepest intrapsychic level available to the patient and working with all the resources the patient possesses and can bring to bear on the problem. Sample modifications to STDP for ill patients may include sharpening the focus, framing the therapy as a holding environment, introducing out-of-session structures for containment, adding out-of-session resources and tasks for learning and reinforcement, offering maintenance returns, changing or supplementing the modality (e.g., individual to group), and extending the contract or making referrals for open-ended psychotherapy when necessary. (For example, it would be cruel and unethical to abandon a seriously ill and deteriorating patient.)

Further Dimensions of Treatment

Throughout the treatment, countertransference responses to Solange were predominantly related to the magnitude of her illness, the extensive fabric of her loss, and her characteristic coping style. It was easy to like her and to admire her brave and endearing qualities. She evoked a protective mothering wish in the therapist, especially in response to her initial overwhelmed state. Anxiety contagion was handled by the clarifying and sorting undertaken early in the process, which reduced both Solange's anxiety and the therapist's anxiety, which was less than conscious at the time. The therapist did become aware of a definite tendency toward identification with Solange's early loss and subsequent "good girl" self-reliance pattern. The awareness could then be put to use by exploring the patient's internal world without confusing Solange's dynamics with her own and without projecting her own needs onto Solange.

It would be easy for an inexperienced therapist to fall into the trap of disliking the father for not helping Solange come to terms with her mother's death. By recognizing the induction, it became possible to help Solange explore her father's discomfort with the expression of feelings other than anger and the impact of the father's style on her through the years. Even in the short time available, Solange developed a more realistic adult appraisal of his strengths and limitations. She was a gratifying patient, because she had a clear and pressing need for psychological help and she was able to make good use of the relationship and the interventions offered. She did not stir the negative countertransference states that some patients stir by being provocative, negative, manipulative, or assaultive. When the treatment ended, the therapist was left with hopeful wishes for Solange's future, tempered by the knowledge that her health remained fragile.

The illness interacted with Solange's world in a strong way by limiting major choices about roles and the life stages ahead of her. Pregnancy would be difficult and would represent a danger to her. This knowledge would necessarily impinge on significant relationships and her choice of a mate. Regarding her history, the similarity of her mother's illness to her own played an important part in Solange's understanding of her illness. Issues about her mother became a vital part of the treatment.

Solange's large family was supportive of her throughout her illness. They were ready to step in as caretakers and to meet her financial needs. Her father was particularly attentive, and she felt the loss of his attention keenly when she became less acutely ill and he became less available. The multigenerational meaning of kidney failure is noteworthy in this family, where the mother died prematurely due to renal failure and the daughter's life became endangered. The father responded to his daughter's crisis by moving toward her. An alternative response to Solange's illness could have occurred if this father had fled from the presence of the disease that took the life of his first wife and the mother of his children. He was not a man who could discuss feelings, but he acted responsively. In an ideal world, family therapy at the time of the mother's death would have been of great help to this family. Although family therapy was not the modality used for Solange, some interventions were made within a family systems framework for her continued work on communications and roles when she returned home to Canada.

Narrative Case Treatment Description

Case Overview

Solange was a 24-year-old French Canadian college graduate, who was referred for psychotherapy during a 4-month stay in the United States, after which she returned to Canada. She was fluent in both French and English. In appearance, she was a slightly overweight attractive young woman who dressed casually. In manner, she was soft-spoken, articulate, and able to form a therapeutic relationship quite readily. The referral source was a personal contact through the National Kidney Foundation in the United States.

Presenting Problem

During the initial evaluation session, Solange's chief complaint was feeling "let down." Her problem was centered around a delayed emotional reaction to a debilitating and life-threatening illness, thrombocytopenic purpura (described below). She was unable to identify the nature of her reaction. During the year of her illness and the following year of her recuperation, she had been oriented toward the intertwined goals of facing each day with courage and getting well. Now that she no longer had to be heroic to survive, she found herself feeling sad, tearful, and somewhat lost, without any goals. She reported feeling overwhelmed and unable to cope with her life effectively.

Background

Solange is the fifth of eight children in a large Roman Catholic family. Her father is a professional man; her mother died at about the time Solange was old enough to begin school. The cause of her mother's death was kidney failure, associated with lupus. Her father remarried, and subsequent family life has provided a stable and reliable environment. A striking note in the family's history is that the father gathered all of the children together at church and told them of their mother's death; after that one occasion, he did not discuss their mother or her death with them.

Toward the end of Solange's senior year at her university, she developed a blood clotting disorder. The disorder is thrombocytopenic purpura, which is a lupus-associated disease similar to the one that took her mother's life. Within 6 weeks, her kidneys failed, due to internal bleeding at the entrance to both kidneys. As a life-preserving measure, she was maintained on renal dialysis, three times a week, for 1 year. During that time, she was febrile, lethargic, and bedridden for the most part. When a kidney became available to her through an international foundation, she elected to have kidney transplant surgery. The transplantation of the new kidney was successful. Three months later, she was able to return to finish her studies and graduate. After a slight initial rejection reaction to the donor kidney, Solange's body tolerated the new kidney well. For the year preceding her psychotherapy, she had been in good health, maintained on a daily regimen of immunosuppressant medication. Her condition necessitates lifelong medical maintenance and follow-up.

Precipitating Event

Approximately 1 month before her initial psychotherapy visit, Solange received news that a friend of hers, a man who also suffered from kidney disease, was ill. They had met originally at their dialysis center and developed a nonintimate but friendly and supportive relationship, as many patients in similar circumstances do. He underwent transplant surgery on the same day she did, with each of them receiving one kidney from the same donor source. They joked about a twinship bond. On Solange's most recent visit to the medical clinic for her monthly follow-up examination, she learned that his system had rejected the transplanted kidney and that he was once again receiving dialysis treatments. This development was extremely unsettling for Solange; she felt terrible for him, and she became increasingly concerned about her own future.

Impression

Solange appeared to have a reactive depression. She was experiencing a truncated and anxious grief reaction to loss. The stressor of illness was a large, intrusive, disturbing presence in her life.

Specifically, she was aware of struggling to face fears about her health in the future and what it would mean to her to lose her transplanted kidney. She was not aware of grieving multiple losses: the loss of time spent ill and tied to dialysis, the loss of a necessary part of her body, the loss of her family's attention after her recovery, or the loss of her mother from a related disease. Initially, she could tell of these events but could not connect her present feelings to her profound losses. The truncating or disconnecting process needed further assessment beyond the first session, but its presence was consistent with her presentation of a denying stoic pattern since early childhood. The stoicism seemed rooted in her family's religious and self-in-family values.

Contract

Psychotherapy would have to be accomplished within a 14-week period because Solange's stay in the United States was time limited. Despite this daunting constraint, she had the focus, the energy, and the desire to work intensively within a short-term context. She was not hampered by vegetative depressive symptoms (i.e., sleeping, eating, or concentration disturbances) that could retard the process. She was willing to commit herself to weekly 50-minute psychotherapy sessions and to call between sessions if necessary.

Course of Treatment

The first stage of treatment involved establishing the therapeutic alliance, identifying the nature of her distress, and helping her to articulate her grief. She responded with great relief to the formulation of the focus: her paramount grief reaction to her losses and her anxiety about her future. The supportive, reflective, and clarifying aspects of the beginning of therapy allowed her to release some of her sadness and anxiety so that she could tolerate better an exploration of the underlying causes of her discomfort. She developed a positive transference, which was somewhat idealizing.

From that point on, the essential task became to distinguish between what was lost and what might be retrievable or added, in order to increase her ability to influence the direction and quality of her life. This "sorting" focus was a task she could undertake successfully. She needed to discover new abilities and to rediscover or reclaim some abilities that had been put aside or temporarily lost. Solange had already painfully acknowledged helplessness over disease that cannot be controlled or predicted. She needed relief from her sense of helplessness and overwhelmed states. The psychologist's early hypothesis concerning her grief was that if she could acknowledge the control (and wishes for control) she does have, then she could acknowledge the losses she could not control, could mourn without shame, and could recover with a reconsolidation within herself.

As a result of exploring areas of loss and areas of control, three interconnected issues emerged that needed to be addressed: (a) her perceptions of her body, (b) her relationship with her present family (especially father and stepmother), and (c) her identification with her mother and her mother's disease. At first, the connections were not clear to either patient or therapist. She seemed to be skipping around topics but was able to allow herself to introduce them in her own way with some encouragement. By the third or fourth session, she was able to move more and more freely between and among the three interconnected areas, and the slightly disjointed quality of the psychotherapy disappeared. The quality of that change was the first clinical evidence available to indicate that integration would be possible and that the truncating process need not be maintained.

Overall, in the middle phase of the treatment, the psychotherapeutic approach involved two basic kinds of interventions to help Solange adapt and take charge of her own adult life:

1. A dynamic process of interpretation and the connection of feelings to central events and personal meanings (especially those related to her body, relationships with family, and identification with mother), and

2. The assignment of out-of-session tasks.

Out-of-session tasks seem to be widely used by therapists to help mobilize a patient's personal resources and to reinforce, by practice, important session learning. In this instance, the tasks were tailored specifically to provide a means for her to test her reactions to others for reality, personal meaning, and distortion (in technical terms, her valences regarding object relations and expectations for self). For example, Solange had many questions, along with much anxiety and resentment, about dietary restrictions necessitated by her illness. During this middle phase, she arranged an appointment with a specialist dietitian and, for the first time, addressed her diet concerns directly.

By the 12th session, the exploration of her losses and the areas for potential control that were related to the losses yielded the following dimensions. She had suffered profound losses—of her health, kidneys, and 2 years of her life; she had gained control over her diet, her career selection (as related to her physical stamina factor), and her decisions about sexual activity in the present and pregnancy in the future. These last two decisions were made in the contexts of her health and of a relationship with a young man.

She had lost the worried and controlling attention that the family paid to her during her illness (especially her father, who had been very distressed by her illness), but she could control her requests for pleasant attention, for example, by initiating social plans with family members during visits. She had lost her mother and longed for her, but she had discovered that she could control her access to information about her mother through other people. Because Solange had viewed her father as the only link to her mother and he would not talk about her, she knew very little about her mother except the cause of her death. She did not even know her mother's birthday. Solange had been at an internal impasse, caught between her wish to know her mother and her wish to protect her father. The perceived need to protect her father had been based on her perception about his omnipotent power and his avoidance of vulnerability. Part of the process of regaining control over her life's direction was to expand the links to her mother to include older siblings, her aunt, and her grandmother. It also involved trusting her own few memories of her mother. She made calls to some of her relatives to talk about her mother, and she visited in person when she returned to Canada briefly for her monthly medical checkup.

One of the most visible changes in Solange occurred when she relinquished her defensive posture of approaching an important person only through an intermediary. She had developed the protective stance after her mother's death, as a reaction formation made necessary by her father's silence about her mother. She believed one must never ask a direct question, especially not of a powerful male authority figure, but must take an indirect route for information or emotional supplies. She had always used her stepmother as a conduit through which to make requests of her father. Regarding her present health concerns, she had never approached her physician, but saved her questions for the medical social worker. As one of her out-of-session tasks, she asked her nephrologist several questions of importance to her about her condition, prescriptions, and quality-of-life decisions; she was pleased with her own assertiveness and relieved by his responsiveness to her.

The psychotherapy moved toward the termination phase. At the beginning of the phase, Solange's positive feelings and newfound confidence were in the ascendancy, whereas negative feelings were quiescent. The depression had lifted. By self-report, she felt able to cope with events as they might arise. She felt more relaxed and no longer wanted to hide, to avoid facing herself and others. She could talk about the possibility of feeling overwhelmed again if her kidney were to fail; however, she believed she would be able to cope if it should happen. Her confidence at this juncture seemed to be a reflection of two dimensions. First, she was experiencing a solid sense of satisfaction and comfort with the level of resolution she had accomplished. Second, she had not yet begun to grapple with feelings that might be associated with the termination of therapy, which involves the loss of present support and also could cause echoes of maternal loss.

Solange demonstrated a widening tolerance for affect, especially negative affect. As she became more assertive, her anger started to emerge. During a telephone conversation with her father, she raised her voice and yelled back when he yelled at her, as he did frequently to all of his children. Apparently, they were both surprised, and her father apologized to her for losing his temper. During another exchange, Solange refused a request made by her stepmother, because she was aware of resenting the intrusive nature of the request.

In session, Solange evaluated the impact on her of the family pattern of expressing anger. She discussed her own anger in more straightforward and direct ways. She was recognizing the family matrix in which the men (father and brothers) may explode and are expected to do so, whereas the women (stepmother and sisters) keep silent and avert their eyes from the men, whom they view as irrational and immensely powerful. This anger work was congruent and important for her, but it was also incomplete, because there was not enough time to work it through before the psychotherapy came to an end.

The psychologist recognized the many possibilities for difficulties in Solange's connection and integration of present anger associated with three sets of experiences: past unacknowledged fury after the death of her mother, loss of her father's attention when he married her stepmother soon afterward, and the loss of her health at an age when asserting independence is important developmentally. It would have been a formidable task in that brief time for her to fully resolve the web that included anger, abandonment, and death themes from the past, present, and the predictable future if her transplanted kidney were to fail. In open-ended long-term psychotherapy, Solange would have been able to weather the necessary storms and live the anger through to integration in the therapy relationship. As it happened, it was not appropriate or possible to arrive at an anger phase in the transference, because there was not a regression to a transference neurosis. In fact, Solange needed a positive experience consciously and in all likelihood also needed to preserve her therapist unconsciously as the good mother with whom she was seeking reunion.

The last tasks were to assess together the work that had been finished and the work that remained to be accomplished in the future and to say good-bye. She felt sad about the ending and wished the therapy could continue. She wavered a bit about leaving, but knew the best path for her was a return to Canada as planned. The therapist supported her choice and her strength. In the final session, Solange tried to mobilize her family's coping style, by telling herself that since the crisis was over and her

depression lifted, there was no reason to coddle herself by wanting to stay. The therapist reminded her that she was entitled to
her wishes, especially when going through a separation, and that
feelings for people are natural, not an aberrant weakness. For
comfort, Solange held on to the positive experience of therapy,
saying she would not forget what the experience had given her
and that she might seek therapy again, especially if she became
ill. She expected to continue her search for information, pictures,
and stories about her mother, feeling strongly the need to do so.
Solange finished her treatment having reached a new level of
adaptation to her illness and her life circumstances.

Summary

We have used the case of Solange to illustrate our hologram of
understanding chronic illness and the psychotherapy of these
patients. Other dimensions may be worth illuminating to
enhance this multiplex hologram. Additional views may be
added to the model as they become available.

It is our hope that the model will help the general psychotherapy practitioner to work with greater effectiveness and to have
more understanding of patients with chronic illness. Furthermore, we hope that more community practitioners will cull their
best primary care experiences and contribute their own views. A
broader, wider, and deeper base of clinical knowledge will
enhance our understanding of the special needs of these patients.
New insight and research from the community setting is essential for integration into the existing and growing scientific base of
psychological and medical research.

Patients need support and psychotherapy in their communities,
near to home. After leaving a big city medical center at the end of
her cancer treatment, one patient remarked, "You're all alone out
here. Everything suddenly stops when you go home. Wham,
there's no transition." As community practitioners, we hear similar versions of her story frequently. Coping with the changes
brought about by chronic illness continues long after the patient
leaves the hospital. Psychotherapy that is targeted at improved
adaptation and coping must be available to meet those needs.

III

Resources

11

A Compendium of Information and Services

Organizations abound. They range from general health agencies to private, thematic groups, and they provide information, support, and services to patients, families, caregivers, health care professionals, and educators. Space limitations prevent a complete listing here. National groups can refer inquirers to a local affiliate or other local resources or groups. All of the organizations listed below offer general medical information. Most provide social services and support groups through local affiliates. Local chapters of national organizations must be contacted directly to pinpoint available services. The toll-free number of the larger organizations often routes callers to the area affiliate; for access to specialized material, the main office number may be more helpful.

Most of the literature mentioned in this section can be ordered through the specific organizations, but some materials are mentioned only as recommendations. Basic information is usually provided free of charge, particularly to patients; in some cases, additional material is available for a small fee (to cover the cost of photocopying and postage). It is a good idea to ask for a publication list and bibliography. Some groups require membership fees in exchange for receiving regular newsletters and updates.

Primarily dedicated to serving patients and their families, many organizations gladly provide information to physicians and other health care providers. Most touch briefly on emotional aspects in their patient-directed literature; a handful have done research into psychosocial issues. Counseling services or material of particular psychosocial interest are noted.

Each listing includes a brief description of the services provided. Contact the organization for more detailed information. To learn about a group with a particular focus not listed here, you may contact one of the general organizations or consult the local telephone directory. An excellent source of information that may be available at a local library is the *Encyclopedia of Associations*, edited by Carolyn A. Fischer and Carol A. Schwartz (published by Gale Research, Inc.). Volume 2 lists organizations under the subjects Health & Medical and Social Welfare.

If you have access to on-line services (e.g., Internet), you can get information almost immediately. Much of the material found on-line comes from the agencies listed here; those with on-line services are so denoted. Additional on-line resources include informal discussion groups. A quick search under "chronic illness" on the Internet yielded nearly 30 resources, more than half of which were discussion groups for patients–caregivers, functioning as support groups. Keep in mind, however, that not all are moderated.

To avoid redundancy, abbreviations have been used to describe common services. Each can stand for any or all of the services designated in the following list and is meant to give a general idea of the services provided.

Abbreviations Used in This Chapter

ADA   Provides information about the Americans With Disabilities Act, compliance, and legal–civil rights; refers to agencies for assistance.

CGV   Caregivers. Provides information and support to caregivers and family.

CT   Clinical trials. Information and referrals to ongoing clinical trials.

EDUC   Education. Advocates educational rights (especially for children); refers to schools and federal–state

	agencies; provides information on special problems–solutions and the Individualized Education Program.
EIP	Early Intervention Program.
EMP	Employment. Advocates employment rights; refers to federal–state agencies and placement programs; networking; job listings.
FIN	Financial assistance or referrals to agencies that provide assistance.
GMI	General medical information (usually brochures discussing diagnosis, treatments, and research).
HCP	Health care professionals (physicians, nurses, others).
ICH	Information clearinghouse; provides medical information, usually from many sources, including medical journal article reprints.
IEP	Individualized Education Plan.
LC	Local chapters–affiliates connected to the national organization that provide social services, referrals, and literature.
LGL	Provides legal advice, assistance, counseling, referrals, or funds.
LIT	Literature (brochures, books, medical article reprints, newsletters, fact sheets, pamphlets, medical journals, monographs, surveys, government reports, and audiovisual materials).
NIH	National Institutes of Health.
OL	On-line services (computer database information).
OT	Occupational therapy.
PAT	Patient.
PCG	Peer counseling groups.
PSY	Psychologist–psychological.
PT	Physical therapy.
REC	Recreational activities: children's camps, athletics, social functions, etc.
RFM	Medical referrals to local physicians, specialists, clinical trials, studies, or specialized medical or other treatment centers.

RFS   Referrals to social services in local areas: practical,
               legal, financial, educational, transportation, counsel-
               ing, physical–occupational–speech therapy, recre-
               ational activities, or government agencies. Also,
               referrals to other, more specific organizations,
               groups, or resources.
SG   Support groups. Primarily governed through local
               chapters or by experienced patients; usually emo-
               tional support, sometimes includes speakers, work-
               shops, or peer counseling, sometimes purely social.
SS   Social Security.
ST   Speech therapy.
STAT   Statistics.
*   May be of special interest to psychotherapists or
               their patients.

Aging

National Council on the Aging
409 3rd Street, SW, 2nd floor, Washington, DC 20024, (202) 479-
   1200/6653
Information and consultation center. Members only. Volunteer
program, retirement, and life planning seminars, EMP, CGV LIT,
RFS, OL, LGL, special needs clothing and equipment. HCP LIT:
abstracts in social gerontology.

Center for the Study of Aging
706 Madison Avenue, Albany, NY 12208, (518) 465-6927
Health professional organization. Programs in mental health.
Consultant services in nutrition, physical and mental fitness,
home care, long-term care, social–health research, training, and
education. Conferences. Library. Book: *Psychology, Motivation
and Programs.*

Beverly Foundation
70 South Lake Avenue, Suite 750, Pasadena, CA 91101, (818) 792-
   2292

Focuses on long-term health care, supportive services and life quality of people with chronic care needs, especially older adults, their families, and caregivers. LIT (behavioral issues in long-term care).

AIDS

Services for AIDS patients and caregivers are provided through ministries, clinical trials, fundraising foundations, special interest groups, health care professional associations, support–social service groups, and legal–political councils. Only the most general AIDS-related organizations are listed below.

CDC National AIDS Clearinghouse
P.O. Box 6003, Rockville, MD 20849-6003, (800) 458-5231, (800) 342-AIDS (CDC national AIDS hotline), (800) TRIALS-A (clinical trial information service), (800) HIV-0440 (treatment information service)
A service of the Centers for Disease Control. GMI on HIV/AIDS for PAT, HCP, educators, and others; RFM, RFS, CT, OL, EMP, LIT. Internet mailbox: aidsinfo@cdcnac.aspensys.com. Referrals to national groups.

National Minority AIDS Council
191 13th Street, NW, Washington, DC 20009, (202) 483-6622
ICH; STAT.

National Association of People with AIDS
1413 K Street, NW, Washington, DC 20005, (202) 898-0414, (202) 789-2222 (AIDS Fax)
GMI; RFS; Bulletin board: NAPWA-LINK.

Alzheimer's Disease

Alzheimer's Association
919 North Michigan Avenue, Suite 1000, Chicago, IL 60611, (312) 335-8700, (800) 272-3900,
Educational programs for HCPs; LC (218 nationwide); STAT; RFM; RFS. *CGV support systems.

Alzheimer's Disease International
12 South Michigan Avenue, Chicago, IL 60603, (312) 335-5777
CGV.

Amputation

For information about athletics and glove and shoe exchanges,
see Disability; Veterans; Cancer; Diabetes.

American Amputee Foundation
P.O. Box 250218 Hillcrest Station, Little Rock, AR 72225, (501)
   666-2523, (501) 666-9540
LGL; FIN, including low-interest loans; rehabilitation, technical,
and scientific information about prosthetics; self-help programs.
*Free PCG to new amputees and families.

Arthritis

Arthritis Foundation
1314 Spring Street, NW, Atlanta, GA 30309, (404) 872-7100, (800)
   283-7800
GMI; advocacy; SG; RFM; RFS; exercise programs; self-help class
teaching active role in self-care (medications, joint protection,
energy conservation, exercise, reduction of pain and depression).
Workshops, conferences. LIT/videos (on coping techniques,
family–psychosocial issues, teachers' and parents' guides, self-
management, pregnancy, sex, medications, and literature for
children); PT; OT; FIN; EMP; EDUC; SS benefits. *Clinical
PSY/occupational therapist on staff.

National Arthritis and Musculoskeletal and Skin
Diseases Information Clearinghouse
P.O. Box AMS, 9000 Rockville Pike, Bethesda, MD 20892, (301)
   495-4484
ICH; LIT; bibliography of resources for children, parents, and
teachers.

Asthma

Asthma and Allergy Foundation of America
1717 Massachusetts Avenue, NW, Suite 305, Washington, DC 20036, (800) 7-ASTHMA

American Lung Association
1740 Broadway, New York, NY 10019-4374, (800) 586-4872

Blindness

Referrals can be given to specific groups that focus on the deaf–blind, veterans, guide dog users, braille proponents, and special interests or careers.

American Council of the Blind
1155 15th Street, NW, Suite 720, Washington, DC 20005, (202) 467-5081, (800) 424-8666
LC, ICH, EMP, FIN, LGL, RFS, REC, scholarships, advocacy. OL information service: (202) 331-1058. Special interest groups. Council of Families with Visual Impairments (parents of blind children: SG). Lists of providers of reading material, product catalogs, computer products, guide dog schools, travel information.

American Foundation for the Blind
11 Penn Plaza, Suite 300, New York, NY 10001, (212) 502-7600, (800) AFB-LINE
CGV, EDUC, LGL, EMP, ADA, OL (Internet, ERIC). LIT on adjustment, aging, attitudes toward blindness, dreams, young children, multiple disabilities, sex, sports, residential schools, kiddie canes, noncane devices, travel, independent living services for older blind, tips for family members, technology; *Journal of Visual Impairment and Blindness* (in print or on ERIC).

National Federation of the Blind

1800 Johnson Street, Baltimore, MD 21230, (410) 659-9314, (800) 638-7518

LC (600 nationwide) CGV, EMP, EDUC, LGL, RFS. Provides *Braille Monitor*, a report on advocacy, self-organization, social concerns, products, and other relevant topics. LIT for parents of blind children and individuals with diabetes; blind rehabilitation referrals; Job Opportunities for the Blind (nationwide listing and referral); scholarships; SS benefits; assessment tests. *Liaison to the American Psychological Association.

Cancer

The following organizations are only a few of the many cancer-related organizations.

American Cancer Society (ACS)

1599 Clifton Road, NE, Atlanta, GA 30329, (404) 320-3333, (800) ACS-2345

GMI, LC (3,300 nationwide), SG, FIN, RFS, REC, LIT, PAT, and HCP education, research: Programs: I Can Cope; Reach to Recovery; CanSurmount; Road to Recovery (transportation); Look Good, Feel Better; Man to Man (prostate cancer: one-on-one visitation, education, and support); children's camps, CanSurmount (one-on-one visitation). New video: *A Significant Journey* (for breast cancer survivors). Ostomy rehabilitation program. Conferences and workshops. Specific information and services are not available at all local units: ask for division contact. HCP LIT: *CA—A Cancer Journal for Clinicians* (bimonthly); *Cancer Facts and Figures* (annual statistical report); *Oncology Social Work—A Clinician's Guide* (Publication No. 3001). *The national ACS established a Behavioral Research Unit. The founding director is Dr. Frank Baker, a clinical psychological researcher. The unit focuses on psychological research related to psychosocial aspects of disease and treatment, lifestyle issues related to onset of cancer and survivors' needs. A few intervention studies are ongoing.

NCI—Cancer Information Service

(800) 4-CANCER (9 A.M.–7 P.M., Mondays–Fridays)
GMI, CT, RFS, LIT. Provides National Cancer Institute material on specific cancers. Publication lists available.
*LIT: *Guide for Black Americans; Taking Time: Support for People With Cancer and the People Who Care About Them*; and publications about disease recurrence, relief from pain, children's eating problems during treatment, talking with children about cancer, chemotherapy, and radiation therapy.
*PDQ (Physician's Data Query), a computer database for retrieval of cancer information, includes current treatment approaches and investigational protocols. The Internet e-mail address is cancernet@icicb.nci.nih.gov (enter the word *HELP* in the BODY section of the mail message). Requests for information about cancer can be faxed to CancerNet at 301-480-8105.
*PAT/physician versions of information from PDQ (e.g., diagnoses, histology, prognosis, citations and abstracts, statements on investigational drugs, treatment summaries) are available from CancerFax at 301-402-5874 (dialed directly from the fax phone).

Candlelighters Childhood Cancer Foundation

7910 Woodmont Avenue, Suite 460, Bethesda, MD 20814-3015,
    (800) 366-2223
LC, SG, CGV, LIT, LGL, RFS, SS, REC, EMP, EDUC. This is the main resource for family members of children or adolescents with cancer; provides parent-to-parent visitation and information about transportation, blood and wig banks, speakers, kids' meetings, and bereavement groups. Workshops. *LIT: educating child with cancer (issues of reentry, cognitive late effects, communication between parents and educators, legal rights); bone marrow transplantation (medical and coping information); leading self-help groups; organizing and maintaining support groups; wish fulfillment organizations; impact on families; role of family friends; support systems; psychosocial needs; socioeconomic considerations in survival; pain management. Publication lists, book reviews. "Back to School" Nite to educate teachers, other parents, and students.

Cancer Care

1180 Avenue of the Americas, New York, NY 10036, (212) 221-3300, (800) 813-HOPE

PAT, CGV, RFS. *Short-term telephone counseling by specially trained social workers with master's degrees (emotional support, problem solving, doctor–patient communication; information on second opinions, home care, transportation, child care, FIN, pain management, access to entitlements, diagnoses and treatment options, fatigue, loss of appetite, etc.). Teleconferencing SG for homebound; bereavement counseling. Annual symposium on pain for social workers and therapists.

Cerebral Palsy

United Cerebral Palsy Associations

1600 L Street, NW, Suite 700, Washington, DC 20036-5602, (800) USA-5UCP

Referrals to LC (which may also be listed in the white pages of local telephone directories). GMI, EMP, EIP, SG, RFS: hospital benefits, housing, child care, supported living.

Chronic Fatigue Syndrome

National Chronic Fatigue Syndrome and Fibromyalgia Association

3521 Broadway, Suite 222, Kansas City, MO 64111, (816) 931-4777

LC (400 nationwide), SG, CT, ADA, OL, GMI (diagnostics, drugs, research updates). LIT: coping, emotions, educational success, guide for schools and teachers, maintaining careers, neuropsychological rehabilitation techniques, SS disability benefits, NICD report. HCP LIT. *Educational audiotapes and videotapes including coping skills for families, friends, patients, and psychological concerns.

CFIDS Association of America, Inc.
P.O. Box 220398, Charlotte, NC 28222-0398, (800) 442-3437, (900)
   896-CFID Information line
GMI, SG, patient-oriented conference, HCP, research news. LIT:
books, journals, back issues of newsletter, media and medical
article reprints, including "The Psychiatric Status of Patients
With the CFS." Audiotapes and videotapes.

Cystic Fibrosis

Cystic Fibrosis Foundation
6931 Arlington Road, Suite 200, Bethesda, MD 20814, (301) 951-
   4422, (800) 344-4823
GMI, CT, research updates, consensus guidelines, and health
care and insurance issues. RFM: 115 care centers affiliated: medical and social patient services, LC, some SG. LIT, FIN.

Deafness

National Information Center on Deafness
Gallaudet University, 800 Florida Avenue, NE, Washington, DC
   20002-3695, (202) 651-5051
GMI and RFS: EMP, EDUC, FIN, LIT for children, parents, and
teachers; assistive devices and hearing aids, communication,
health, and mental health (including booklets about deaf substance abusers). *The Community Counseling and Mental
Health Clinic (202-651-6083), a training, research, and service
center, serves deaf and hard of hearing people and their families
throughout the country.

National Association of the Deaf
814 Thayer Avenue, Silver Spring, MD 20910, (301) 587-1788,
   TTY: (301) 587-1789
ICH, LGL, RFS, EMP, EDUC, youth programs, rehabilitation,
lobbying, bookstore, *Mental Health Services for Deaf People* (directory of programs and services).

Self-Help for Hard of Hearing People, Inc.
7910 Woodmont Avenue, Suite 1200, Bethesda, MD 20814, (301)
   657-2248, TTY: (301) 657-2249
LC, SG, LIT, assistive devices, alternative communication skills
programs. Coping strategies workshop. CGV, ADA, LGL,
EDUC, EMP, STAT, OL (GEnie bulletin board). PSY LIT:
Manual for Mental Health Professionals; other items dealing with
feelings–behavior, anger, stress, sex, substance abuse, hearing
aids, denial, progressive loss, early–mild loss, and personal and
social considerations.

American Deafness and Rehabilitation Association (ADARA)
P.O. Box 251554, Little Rock, AR 72225, (501) 868-8850
LC, RFS, rehabilitation. OL e-mail: ADARA or ADARA.Board.
Special interest sections (including mental health, chemical
dependency, and vocational placement); *Journal of ADARA*
(research findings, mental health, social services).

Diabetes

National Diabetes Information Clearinghouse
1 Information Way, Bethesda, MD 20892-3560, (800) 496-4000
   (NIH)
A service of the National Institute of Diabetes, Digestive and
Kidney Disease (a branch of NIH) ICH. GMI, OL. Directory of
organizations, resources. Diagnosis, research, treatment, dental
tips, pregnancy, control, and complications. For HCP, STAT on
Hispanics, Native Americans, African Americans.

American Diabetes Association
National Center, P.O. Box 25757, 1660 Duke Street, Alexandria,
   VA 22314, (703) 549-1500, (800) 232-3472
GMI, LC, SG, REC. HCP educational materials and programs.
Research updates. LIT: self-care, cookbooks, nutrition, preg-
nancy, children's books.

Juvenile Diabetes Foundation International

432 Park Avenue South, New York, NY 10016-8013, (212) 785-
9500, (800) JDF-CURE
LC, SG, RFS. *Counseling for parents and children (most of it in
the medical–nutritional vein, because of the nature of disease);
seminars; discussion groups.

Joslin Diabetes Center

1 Joslin Place, Boston, MA 02215, (617) 732-2400
Research and treatment unit. STAT on grants for research.
Specialized education programs for HCP. Barbara Anderson, the
chair of the Behavioral Medicine and Psychology Council of the
American Diabetes Association, states that most of the psychological research–intervention work is with juveniles and the
impact on the family as a whole. Suggested reading: *Psyching
Out Diabetes: A Positive Approach to Your Negative Emotions*, by R.
Rubin, J. Bierman, and J. Toohey, is available through Dr. Rubin
(500 W. University Parkway, Suite 1-M, Baltimore, MD 21210;
also *Diabetes: Caring for Your Emotions as Well as Your Health*, by J.
Edelwich and B. Brodsky (an excellent bibliography that
includes many children's books).

Digestive and Kidney Disease

National Digestive Diseases Information Clearinghouse

2 Information Way, Bethesda, MD 20892-3570 (800) 496-4000
(NIH)
A service of the National Institute of Diabetes and Digestive and
Kidney Diseases, part of NIH. GMI on specific diseases and conditions includes symptoms, treatments, resources, reading lists,
research citations. Networking, referrals. Directory of organizations, LIT for HCP/PAT, STAT. Covers kidney disease, cys-
titis, urinary tract infections, prostate disease, ulcers, gallstones,
Crohn's, cirrhosis, colitis, diverticulitis, irritable bowel syndrome, hepatitis, celiac disease, lupus nephritis, impotence, kidney stones, incontinence, and transplants. Publications include
Kidney Transplantation and Psychological Factors (March 1995),
available from the Combined Health Information Database.

National Kidney Foundation, Inc.

30 East 33rd Street, Suite 1100, New York, NY 10016, (212) 889-
2210, (800) 622-9010
Central office conducts research. LC conduct patient services,
including drug banks, transportation, early screening, seminars.
GMI, RFM, RFS.

American Kidney Fund

6110 Executive Boulevard, Suite 1010, Rockville, MD 20852, (301)
881-3052, (800) 638-8299
Provides direct FIN; supports dialysis center emergency funds;
GMI (telephone line and pamphlets); regional conferences for
HCP.

American Association of Kidney Patients

100 South Ashley Drive, Suite 280, Tampa, FL 33602, (813) 223-
7099, (800) 749-2257
Serves patients and families coping with the physical and emotional effects of kidney disease.

Psychonephrology Foundation

c/o New York Medical College, Psychiatric Institute, Valhalla,
NY 10595, (914) 285-8424
Conducts conferences devoted to psychological issues surround-
ing patients with kidney failure. LIT: *Psychological Factors in
Hemodialysis and Transplantation; Psychological Problems in Kidney
Failure and Their Treatment.*

American Foundation for Urologic Disease

300 West Pratt Street, Suite 401, Baltimore, MD 21201, (800) 242-
2383, (410) 727-2908

Disability

National Information Center for Children and Youth with Disability

P.O. Box 1492, Washington, DC 20013-1492, (800) 695-0285
(voice/TT), (202) 884-8200 (voice/TT)

Information on the following conditions: autism, cerebral palsy, deafness, Down's syndrome, epilepsy, attention deficit disorder, visual impairments. Rare syndrome file. ICH, GMI, CGV, EDUC, ADA, FIN, OL, RFS. LIT: sibling issues, education, sexuality, estate planning, assessment tests, mental health, behavior management (children's literature also available). No medical staff. Medical texts. Internet address: nichcy@aed.org. SpecialNet User Name: NICHCY.

Clearinghouse on Disability Information

U.S. Department of Education, Office of Special Education and Rehabilitative Services, 400 Maryland Avenue, SW, Switzer Building, Room 3132, Washington, DC 20202-2524, (202) 205-8241

Information on federally funded programs and legislation affecting the disabled community. RFS, LGL, EDUC, federal benefits, medical services.

National Easter Seal Society

230 West Monroe, Chicago, IL 60606, (312) 726-6200

Disabilities served: stroke, head trauma, cerebral palsy, developmental disability, hearing disorders, polio, muscular dystrophy, Alzheimer's and others. LC (500 nationwide) serving children with disabilities and their parents. Support services: advocacy, PT, OT, speech therapy and language therapy, vocational evaluation and training, computer-assisted technological training, REC. Loans equipment. Disability awareness (for teachers and other children), ADA, employer sensitivity. Catalog of print and audiovisual resources. Internet address: http://www.seals.com.

American Council on Education Heath Resource Directory

The Heath Resource Center, One Dupont Circle, Suite 800, Washington, DC 20036-1193, (202) 939-9320

Resource directory for those with disabilities and their families and advocates, highlighting organizations that focus on advocacy, awareness, architectural access, education and career access, literacy, family support, the arts, employment, independent living, rehabilitation, legal assistance (ADA).

Commission on Mental and Physical Disability Law
c/o American Bar Association, 740 15th Street, NW, Washington, DC 20005-1009, (202) 662-1570
Primarily geared toward attorneys, providing (for a fee) information on court decisions, legislation, and administrative developments affecting people with mental and physical disabilities. Life services planning. LGL research available. Publications: *The ADA and People with Mental Illness, ADA Manual, Right to Refuse Antipsychotic Medication, Psychiatric Care and Substitute Consent,* as well as others covering AIDS/HIV, the elderly, and guardianship issues.

Epilepsy

Epilepsy Foundation of America
4351 Garden City Drive, Landover, MD 20785, (301) 459-3700, (800) EFA-1000
LC (85 nationwide) provide assistance and counseling. GMI, LGL, RFM, RFS, EMP, EDUC, LIT: book and video catalog; recommended reading; article reprints: "Cognitive and Psychosocial Effects of Epilepsy on Adults"; "Psychosocial Consequences of Epilepsy"; "Assessment of Psychosocial and Emotional Factors in Epilepsy"; "The Quality of Life of Patients with Epilepsy." STAT. Social, rehabilitation, advocacy, and self-help programs. School Alert (a national educational program for schools); mail-order pharmacy. *Assistance and counseling provided through LC.

Epilepsy Concern Service Group
1282 Wynnewood Drive, West Palm Beach, FL 33417, (407) 683-0044
Starts and maintains self-help groups (self-governed). Includes groups for friends and loved ones. Long Distance Friends Program (communicate by letter or tape). Provides group leader training. Epilepsy Concern Starter Kit available to those wishing to organize a community group.

Gulf War Syndrome

Information on Gulf War Syndrome is hard to obtain. The Department of Defense has a Persian Gulf Conflict Hotline: Individuals with symptoms may call (800) 796-9699 to register and set up an examination. Doctors and others who witness symptoms should report that information to (800) 472-6719. A study conducted in December 1994 provides the most recent (and perhaps the only) information available on the syndrome at press time; for a copy of the study, call the Defense Department's Public Communications Department at (703) 697-5737. No separate support groups or service organizations specific to this syndrome were found.

Disabled American Veterans
National Service and Legislative Headquarters, 807 Maine
   Avenue, SW, Washington, DC 20024, (202) 554-3501
Primarily concerned with getting compensation claims adjudicated for veterans. Aid to veterans of Gulf War. RFM, GMI.

American Veterans Committee
6309 Bannockburn Drive, Bethesda, MD 20817, (301) 320-6490
Services offered to Gulf War veterans as well as others.

American Service Veterans Association
3955 Denlinger Road, Dayton, OH 45426-2329, (513) 837-0498
Counseling and social service programs for members and families.

National Veterans Association
P.O. Box 43, Mohnton, PA 19540, (610) 374-0177
Special interest in Persian Gulf and Vietnam veterans; advocates for victims of Agent Orange. Psychosocial services, SG, medical and legal library. *Compiling list of psychologists who handle medical cases.

Regular Veterans Association of the United States
RVA Building 217, 2470 Cardinal Loop, Del Valle, TX 78617,
   (817) 284-4388

Service programs through the Veterans Administration; hospital programs; benefits, rehabilitation, EMP.

Headache

National Headache Foundation
5252 North Western Avenue, Chicago, IL 60625, (312) 878-7715, (800) 843-2256
SG. ICH on types, causes and treatment, drugs, hormonal triggers, effects of diet, research studies and updates, stress reduction, traveling. Book reviews, relaxation tapes. *Provides advice on talking to physicians.

Heart Disease

American Heart Association
7272 Greenville Avenue, Dallas, TX 75231-4596, (800) 242-1793
LC (ext. 8721). GMI: cardiovascular disease, stroke, hypertension, diabetes. Research, education, RFS. Many journals. Copies of two articles from the journal *Circulation* are available on request: "Depression and 18-month Prognosis after Myocardial Infarction" and "Triggering of Acute Myocardial Infarction Onset by Episodes of Anger."

Heart Disease Research Foundation
50 Court Street, Brooklyn, NY 11201, (718) 649-6210
Information about cardiovascular disease (prevention, diagnosis, medicosocial problems, multidisciplinary treatment approach). Acupuncture and electrotherapeutics. Effects of personality factors and exercise on the disease.

Hemophilia

National Hemophilia Foundation
110 Greene Street, Suite 303, New York, NY 10012, (212) 219-8180, (800) 424-2634

GMI for HCP, PAT. LC, RFM, RFS, REC, FIN, LGL. Special interest in HIV/AIDS. Newsletters: "NHF Community Alert"; "HANDI Quarterly"; "Nursing Network/Psychosocial News." Resource list, bibliography, LIT: pain control, coping, employment issues, gene therapy, child care, sports, sex, pregnancy, nutrition, PT, self-hypnosis, relaxation and visualization, drugs, carrier testing, parenting issues, children's books, bereavement. "Prevention of Social and Emotional Problems in Boys with Hemophilia." *Directory of hemophilia psychosocial professionals.

Huntington's Disease

Huntington's Disease Society of America
140 West 22nd Street, 6th Floor, New York, NY 10011-2420, (212) 242-1968, (800) 345-4372
GMI for PAT, CGV. Social, economic, and emotional issues; research progress updates. Crisis intervention. SG, FIN, LGL. LIT: practical hints for CGV; daily living–care manuals; PT, OT; nutrition/feeding; juvenile/teens; "Understanding Behavioral Changes in HD"; "Huntington's Chorea: Its Impact on the Spouse." *Psychosocial articles: "Living with the Characterologically Altered Brain-injured Patient"; "Families with HD: Psychologic and Social Treatment"; "Telling the Children"; "Social Work with Victims of HD"; "The Adolescent's Reaction to Chronic Illness of a Parent: Some Implications for Family Counseling"; "Suicide and HD"; "Behavioral and Sexual Problems in HD"; "Living through Grief." Videos are available on caring guides, profiles, communication strategies, overviews.

Hypertension

National Hypertension Association, Inc.
324 East 30th Street, New York, NY 10016, (212) 889-3557
GMI. LIT: medical tips, preventive measures, recipes, behavioral therapies, cholesterol, drugs, obesity, nutrition and diet, smoking, stress and physical activity. STAT. Research.

Article reprints. The association has an information program with the National High Blood Pressure Education Program in Washington (1-800-575-WELL).

Kidney Disease

See Digestive and Kidney Disease.

Liver Disease

See also Digestive and Kidney Disease.

American Liver Foundation
1425 Pompton Avenue, Cedar Grove, NJ 07009, (201) 256-2550, (800) 223-0179
Covers liver disease, hepatitis, gallbladder disease. SG, RFM.

Lupus

Lupus Foundation of America
4 Research Place, Suite 180, Rockville, MD 20850-3226, (301) 670-9292, (800) 558-0121
LC (500 nationwide). GMI; SG; RFM; RFS. Hospital visits. Professional education, physician handbook. Publications that discuss psychosocial issues and daily living include "Coping with Lupus," "Sick and Tired of Being Sick and Tired," and "We Are Not Alone: Learning to Live with Chronic Illness," and *The Disease and Its Patients* by Jon Russell.

The American Lupus Society
260 Maple Court, No. 123, Ventura, CA 93003, (805) 339-0443, (800) 331-1802
GMI, LC, SG, LIT. Pamphlet: *So Now You Have Lupus* (discusses psychological corticosteroid effects, sexuality, self-image, depression, stress).

Lyme Disease

Lyme Disease Foundation
1 Financial Plaza, 18th Floor, Hartford, CT 06103, (203) 525-2000, (800) 886-LYME
LC (200 nationwide). SG, RFM, RFS, medical seminars. Maintains registry of infected pregnant women and congenital cases.

Minority Health

Covers health issues of minorities, including diabetes, heart disease, AIDS, hypertension, tuberculosis, lupus, and gallbladder disease.

Office of Minority Health Resource Center
P.O. Box 37337, Washington, DC 20013-7337, (800) 444-6472
An office of the U.S. Department of Health and Human Services. Provides information on health issues and organizations and individuals working in minority health professions. Fact sheets, RFS, health materials resource lists.

Sickle Cell Disease Association of America
200 Corporate Pointe, Suite 495, Culver City, CA 90230-7633, (800) 421-8453
LC, EDUC, REC. Counselor training; seminars and workshops; blood banks; screening/testing; tutorial services; vocational rehabilitation. LIT. Home study kit for families. Video. Guide to programs and services.

National Asian Pacific Center on Aging
Melbourne Tower, 1511 3rd Avenue, Suite 914, Seattle, WA 98101, (206) 624-1221
STAT. Registry of services. Health issues of Asian Pacific elderly. Research and document family and community support systems. EMP. Library's extensive bibliography encompasses additional subjects: hypertension, cancer, cardiovascular risk, renal disease, stress, social and psychological perspectives, depression, suicide, need patterns, life satisfactions.

Multiple Sclerosis

National Multiple Sclerosis Society
733 3rd Avenue, New York, NY 10017, (212) 986-3240, (800)
　FIGHT-MS
LC, GMI, SG, RFS, RFM, LGL, STAT; OL. Library. LIT: journal
reprints, such as "Cognitive Dysfunction in MS: Impact on
Employment and Social Functioning"; "Psychosocial Adjustment
in MS"; "Effects of MS on Occupational and Career Patterns."
HCP bibliography: neurobehavioral aspects, mental disorders
and cognitive deficits, sexual concerns, guides for families.

Multiple Sclerosis Foundation, Inc.
6350 North Andrews Avenue, Fort Lauderdale, FL 33309, (305)
　776-6805, (800) 441-7055
LC, SG, GMI, RFS, RFM, research updates, health care options.
Suggested reading list: alternative medicine approaches and
symptom management, relaxation techniques, diet and nutrition, exercise. *One-on-one telephone support.

Muscular Dystrophy

Muscular Dystrophy Association
3300 East Sunrise Drive, Tucson, AZ 85718, (602) 529-2000
Clinics provide comprehensive medical services, assistance with
purchase and repair of wheelchairs, PT, OT, and respiratory
therapy, REC, transportation assistance. GMI LIT, audiovisual
materials on the latest research developments. FIN, SG. Genetic
counseling.

Myasthenia Gravis

Myasthenia Gravis Foundation of America, Inc.
222 South Riverside Plaza, Suite 1540, Chicago, IL 60606, (800)
　541-5454
LC, SG, PCG, GMI. *Some telephone support for newly diagnosed patients. LIT for PAT and HCP. They will discuss the

latest treatment options (drugs, surgery, plasmapheresis) and send information, but they do not give medical advice. Mail-order prescription service. Drug interactions. Fighting fatigue; daily living tips. Coping videotape. Educational seminars. *Foundation staff are trying to compile a psychosocial information and referral list and wish to hear from psychologists who treat individuals with chronic illnesses.

Neurofibromatosis

National Neurofibromatosis Foundation
95 Pine Street, 16th Floor, New York, NY 10005, (800) 323-7938
LC (26 nationwide), SG. GMI, RFM, LIT: learning disabilities, psychosocial aspects. OL: http://www.neurofibromatosis.org or http://www.nf.org.

Neurofibromatosis, Inc.
8855 Annapolis Road, Suite 110, Lanham, MD 20706-2924, (301) 577-8984, (800) 942-6825
RFS, PCG, RFM, RFS, LIT. Research updates, medical journal article reprints. Conferences for families/CGV. Networking of voluntary health organizations. Pen pal service for deafened adults. Referrals to SG. Newsletter. LIT: *Psychosocial Aspects of Appearance in Neurofibromatosis,* by Sarah Ellis; "Impact of NF on the Family," by Mary Ann Wilson and Felice Yahr, taken from *Neurofibromatosis: A Handbook for Patients, Families, and Health-Care Professionals* (Thieme Publishers, 1990).

Ostomy

United Ostomy Association
36 Executive Park, Suite 120, Irvine, CA 92714, (714) 660-8624, (800) 826-0826
LC (700 nationwide), SG, GMI, RFS, LIT. *Psychological support and practical information; sponsors visiting program; support of families; advocacy. Patient visiting service: trained and certified

visitors preoperative and postoperative. Some affiliates have trained spouse visitors. Parents of Ostomy Children networks. Youth Rally (12–17-year-olds): hygiene, sexuality, self-care. LIT on general information, care and management, children (including a 90-page resource book for parents of children with disabilities and special care needs), sexuality (including a gay and lesbian brochure), book on coping with ostomy.

Pain

National Chronic Pain Outreach Association
7979 Old Georgetown Road, Suite 100, Bethesda, MD 20814-2429, (301) 652-4948
ICH. GMI: chronic pain and its management options. SG, RFM, RFS. LIT: coping tips, resources, breathing, massage, stress, neuropathy, fibromyalgia, travel, depression, anger, doctor–patient communication, mind–body dilemma, SS, acupuncture, sex, biofeedback, insurance, drug therapy, affirmation–visualization, self-hypnosis, effects on family.

American Pain Society
5700 Old Orchard Road, 1st Floor, Skokie, IL 60077-1024, (708) 966-5595
Provides information on acute pain, cancer pain; journal, *Pain Facilities Directory*.

Parkinsonism

National Parkinson Foundation
1501 NW 9th Avenue, Miami, FL 33136, (305) 547-6666
LC; SG. LIT for HCP, PAT. LIT: Emotional issues—attitudes and adaptations; practical advice. "Practical Pointers for Parkinsonians" (brochure) offers specific practical tips and products. Educational programs. "Parkinson Report" (quarterly): research updates, surgical and pharmacological therapies; addresses

specific problems and gives suggestions (sleep changes, dietary–feeding concerns), patient perspectives–inspirational stories, driving, travel. Information on new research: fetal tissue transplants.

American Parkinson Disease Association

60 Bay Street, Suite 401, Staten Island, NY 10301, (718) 981-8001, (800) 223-APDA

GMI, LC (90 nationwide), SG (500 nationwide), LIT. Educational symposia and conferences for HCP, PAT, CGV. Supports research.

Prostate Disease

American Prostate Association

P.O. Box 4206, Silver Spring, MD 20914, (301) 384-9405

GMI (prostatitis, cancer, noncancerous enlargement) and PAT support.

Stroke

National Stroke Association

8480 East Orchard Road, Suite 1000, Englewood, CO 80111, (303) 771-1700, (800) STROKES

LC, GMI, RFS, LIT (prevention, rehabilitation, resocialization, research). Medical staff to answer questions, clinical updates. Practical information for poststroke rehabilitation, adjustment. Will refer to local stroke club, SG. LIT for HCP/PAT: emotional aspects, communication difficulties–suggestions, home–work adaptations, rehabilitation guidelines and resources, depression, diet, research updates. Newsletter, journal.

Stroke Clubs International

805 12th Street, Galveston, TX 77550, (409) 762-1022

LC (more than 800 nationwide), each with its own agenda. Some SG, some social.

National Aphasia Association
P.O. Box 1887, Murray Hill Station, New York, NY 10156, (800)
   922-4622
GMI, RFS, LGL, LIT, CGV. Bibliographies: psychosocial aspects,
evaluation and treatment. Referrals to community groups.

Veterans

See Blindness, Disability, Gulf War Syndrome.

National Amputation Foundation
73 Church Street, Malverne, NY 11565, (516) 887-3600
For nonveterans and veterans with service-connected amputation. EMP, LGL, social, and mental rehabilitation. Social activities, psychological aid; prosthetic center, including training in
use of devices.

Miscellaneous

Accent on Information
P.O. Box 700, Bloomington, IL 61702, (309) 378-2961
Information searches are provided (for a nominal fee) on daily
care, products and devices for disabled persons. *Buyer's Guide*
lists equipment and devices.

Agency for Health Care Policy and Research
U.S. Department of Health and Human Services, Public Health
   Service, P.O. Box 8547, Silver Spring, MD 20907, (800) 358-9295
Free publications clearinghouse. GMI covers diabetes, depression, stroke rehabilitation, ulcers, sickle cell disease, cancer pain,
heart failure, early HIV infection, elderly, and long-term care,
some information on children's health care. Patient outcomes
research. Clinical practice guidelines for physicians and patients.
24-hour InstantFAX: (301) 594-2800 (to order publications: use
fax phone handset, press 1 at prompt, follow prompts to get

publication number and place an order). STAT. National surveys, article reprints.

American Self-Help Clearinghouse
St. Clares-Riverside Medical Center, Denville, NJ 07834, (201) 625-7101
Call for name and number of state or local organization: information and assistance on local self-help groups. Callers may request *Self-Help Sourcebook*.

Association for the Care of Children's Health
7910 Woodmont Avenue, Suite 300, Bethesda, MD 20814, (301) 654-6549
LIT focusing on the needs of disabled or chronically ill children and their families; particular emphasis on psychosocial issues, developmental support, family-centered care; includes children's books, material about and for fathers. Videos. Resource catalog. Directory of state programs.

Center for Coping with Chronic Conditions
2268 Hempstead Turnpike, East Meadow, NY 11554, (516) 735-2080
LIT topics: coping with anger, guilt; effects of childhood illness on siblings.

Haworth Press
10 Alice Street, Binghamton, NY, (607) 722-5857, (800) 342-9678 (to place orders)
Publisher of journals and books on psychosocial oncology, chemotherapy, OT, PT, pain, grief, AIDS, geriatric long-term care, sexuality and disabilities, terminal care, chronic fatigue syndrome, mental health subjects. Call for catalogs.

Kids on the Block
9385 C Gerwig Lane, Columbia, MD 21046, (301) 290-9095, (800) 368-KIDS
Performing arts puppet show, in which characters have variety of handicaps (available in 49 states).

MedicAlert Tags

(800) 432-5378

A nonprofit foundation that distributes bracelets and necklaces engraved with wearer's personal medical information (e.g., drug allergies, chronic diseases), widely recognized by medical and emergency personnel.

National Association of Private Schools for Exceptional Children

1625 I Street, NW, Suite 506, Washington, DC 20006, (202) 223-2192

Newsletter and directory of private schools for children with special needs.

National Center for Health Statistics

Division of Public Health Service, Hyattsville, MD, (301) 436-8500

"Current Estimates from the National Health Interview Survey 1993," Series 10 #190. Acute and chronic conditions, breakdown by race, age, and gender; diabetes; heart disease; kidney disease. General medical and statistical information. Available at government depository libraries, or from the Government Printing Office, stock #017-022-01-27-91. Telephone: (202) 512-1800.

National Institutes of Health

9000 Rockville Pike, Bethesda, MD 20892, (800) 496-4000, (301) 496-8188

Can connect callers directly to any of 26 institutes, including those dealing with cancer; human genome research; eye, heart, lung, and blood diseases; aging; allergy and infectious diseases; arthritis; musculoskeletal and skin diseases; child health and human development; deafness and other communication disorders; diabetes and digestive and kidney diseases; mental health; neurological disorders and stroke; alternative medicine; women's health. GMI; often can provide a list of referrals to patient social service groups. OL SysOp: (301) 496-6610 (voice), (301) 402-1434 (fax). NIH has a bulletin board system: (301) 480-5144 (Maryland callers) or (800) NIH-BBS1 (all others). Through Internet, use FedWorld BBS; Telnet address is fedworld.gov or 192.239.92.201;

the FTP address is ftp.fedworld.gov or 192.239.92.205. BBS is #127 on the FedWorld list of systems. *Combined Health Information Database is an online reference service for health educators. Available through NIH and affiliates. Access through Ovid Online. Available through CDP Online (some libraries subscribe).

National Lekotek Center
2100 Ridge Avenue, Evanston, IL 60204
Toy lending services, play sessions, and support for children with special needs and families are provided by 48 centers in U.S.

National Self-Help Clearinghouse
25 West 43rd Street, Room 620, New York, NY 10036-7406, (212) 354-8525
ICH. RFS. Research and training activities.

Sibling Information Network
991 Main Street, Suite 3A, East Hartford, CT 06108, (203) 282-7050
For siblings of people with disabilities. RFS. Family issues. LIT, newsletter.

Siblings for Significant Change
823 United Nations Plaza, Room 808, New York, NY 10017, (212) 420-0776
Information and referral services, LGL, counseling, community education.

Specialnet
GTE Education Services, Inc., 2021 K Street, NW, Suite 215, Washington, DC 20006, (202) 835-7300
Computer network offers support for families of children with disabilities.

The Well Spouse Foundation
P.O. Box 801, New York, NY 10023, (212) 644-1241, (800) 838-0879
Private membership organization. Support for spouses or partners of chronically ill or disabled. Newsletter. SG, round-robin

letter writing, personal outreach, annual conference, continued support for bereaved.

State Sources

Developmental Disabilities Council, Dept. of Community Affairs, Dept. of Education/Special Education, Dept. of Health, Dept. of Human Services, Dept. of Labor, Dept. of Law & Public Safety, Dept. of the Public Advocate (or Protection and Advocacy Agency), Dept. of Transportation, State Mental Health Agency, State Mental Health Representative for Children and Youth, State Vocational Rehabilitation Agency, Early Intervention Program (through Special Child Health Services), State Agency for the Visually Impaired.

References

Medical

Berkow, R., & Fletcher, A. (Eds.). (1992). *The Merck manual of diagnosis and therapy* (16th ed.). Rahway, NJ: Merck & Co.
A small medical handbook of information by name of disease, with limited, clear, descriptive, and statistical information that can be understood by nonmedical persons.

Griffith, H.W., & Dambro, M.R. (1994). *The 5-minute clinical consult* (2nd ed.). Philadelphia: Lea & Febiger.
An outstanding synopsis of diseases, concisely organized to give basic medical information. It includes appropriate resources for further information for each disease.

Margolis, S., & Moses, H. (1992). *Johns Hopkins medical handbook.* New York: Rebus.
Briefly discusses 100 major medical disorders common to people over 50, with a directory to leading teaching hospitals, research organizations, treatment centers, and support groups.

Thoene, J.G. (1995). *Physician's guide to rare diseases* (2nd ed.). Montvale, NJ: Dowden.
Concisely describes outcome, process, etiology, and treatment of rare diseases. Gives brief signs and symptoms and lists specific resources for each disease.

Wyngaarden, J.B., Smith, L.H., & Bennett, J.C. (Eds.). (1992). *Cecil textbook of medicine* (19th ed.). Philadelphia: W.B. Saunders.
A comprehensive medical text that gives extensive detail about disease processes, pathophysiology, treatments, etiology, and symptoms.

Young, M.T., & Wingerson, L. (Eds.). (1995). *1996 medical outcomes and guidelines sourcebook.* New York: Faulkner & Gray.
A progress report and resource guide on medical outcomes, research, and practice guidelines that will increasingly affect patients as managed care and medical economics in general seek to limit many types of treatments. Alternative treatments as well as mainstream practices are examined. The *Sourcebook* will be updated periodically.

Psychological

American Cancer Society. (1993). *Americans with Disabilities Act: Legal protection for cancer patients against employment discrimination.* Atlanta, GA: Author.

American Psychiatric Association. (1994). *Diagnostic and statistical manual of mental disorders* (4th ed.). Washington, DC: Author.

Bains, S. (1990, November 10). Many holograms multiply data storage. *New Scientist, 128*, 28.

Bellak, L., & Small, L. (1977). *Emergency psychotherapy and brief psychotherapy* (2nd ed.). New York: Grune & Stratton.

Blos, P. (1967). The second individuation process of adolescence. *Psychoanalytic Study of the Child, 22*, 162–186.

Broadhead, W.E., Kaplan, B.H., Jones, S.A., Wagner, E.H., Schoenback, V.J., Grimson, R., Heyden, S., Tiblin, G., & Gehlback, S.H. (1983). The epidemiologic evidence for a relationship between social support and health. *American Journal of Epidemiology, 117*, 521–537.

Cadman, D., Boyle, M., Szatmari, P., & Offord, D.R. (1987). Chronic illness, disability, and mental and social well-being: Findings of the Ontario child health study. *Pediatrics, 79*, 805–813.

Candlelighters Childhood Cancer Foundation. (1993). *Introduction to the Americans with Disabilities Act: A guide for families of children with cancer and survivors of childhood cancer*. Bethesda, MD: Author.

Combrinck-Graham, L. (1985). A developmental model for family systems. *Family Process, 24*, 139–150.

Czyzewski, D. (1988). Stress management in diabetes mellitus. In M.L. Russell (Ed.), *Stress management for chronic disease* (pp. 270–289). Elmsford, NY: Pergamon.

Deffenbacher, J., Demm, P., & Brandon, A. (1986). High general anger: Correlates and treatment. *Behavior Research and Therapy, 24*, 481–489.

Dell Orto, A.E. (1988). Respite care: A vehicle for hope, the buffer against desperation. In P.W. Power, A.E. Dell Orto, & M.B. Gibbons (Eds.), *Family interventions throughout chronic illness and disability* (pp. 265–280). New York: Springer.

Drell, M.J., Siegel, C.H., & Gaensbauer, T.J. (1993). Post-traumatic stress disorder. In C. Zeanah (Ed.), *Handbook of infant mental health* (pp. 291–304). New York: Guilford Press.

Engel, G.L. (1980, May). The clinical application of the biopsychosocial model. *The American Journal of Psychiatry, 137*, 535–544.

Erikson, E. (1963). *Childhood and society* (2nd ed.). New York: Norton.

Falvo, D.R. (1991). *Medical and psychosocial aspects of chronic illness and disability*. Gaithersburg, MD: Aspen.

Flegenheimer, W. (1982). *Techniques of brief psychotherapy*. New York: Basic Books.

Funch, D.P., & Marshall, J. (1983). The role of stress, social support and age in survival from breast cancer. *Journal of Psychosomatic Research, 27*(1), 77–83.

Goldstein, V., Regnery, G., & Wellin, C. (1981, January). Caretaker's role in fatigue. *Nursing Outlook*, 24–30.

Goodheart, C.D. (1989). Short-term dynamic psychotherapy with difficult clients. In P.A. Keller & S.R. Heyman (Eds.), *Innovations in clinical practice: A source book* (pp. 15–26). Sarasota, FL: Professional Resource Exchange.

Haber, S. (Ed.). (1995). *Breast cancer: A psychological treatment manual*. New York: Springer.

Harpham, W. (1994). *After cancer: A guide to your new life.* New York: Norton.

Hecht, J. (1988, February 4). Holography rides the wavefront. *New Scientist, 117,* 59.

Herek, G.M. (1990). Illness, stigma, and AIDS. In P.T. Costa, Jr., & G.R. VandenBos (Eds.), *Psychological aspects of serious illness: Chronic conditions, fatal diseases, and clinical care* (pp. 107–144). Washington, DC: American Psychological Association.

Holland, J.C., & Rowland, J.H. (Eds.). (1989). *Handbook of psychooncology: Psychological care of the patient with cancer.* New York: Oxford University Press.

Horowitz, M. (1992). *Stress response syndromes* (2nd ed.). Northvale, NJ: Jason Aronson.

Houghton Mifflin. (1993). *The American heritage college dictionary* (3rd ed.). Boston: Author.

Hymovich, D.P., & Hagopian, G.A. (1992). *Chronic illness in children and adults: A psychosocial approach.* Philadelphia: W.B. Saunders.

Justice, B. (1988). Stress, coping, and health outcomes. In M.L. Russell (Ed.), *Stress management for chronic disease* (pp. 14–29). Elmsford, NY: Pergamon.

Kalff, D. (1980). *Sandplay/A psychotherapeutic approach to the psyche.* Boston: Sigo.

Kelly-Hayes, M., Wolf, P.A., Kannel, W.B., Sytkowski, D., D'Agostino, R.B., & Gresham, G.E. (1988). Factors influencing survival and need for institutionalization following stroke: The Framingham study. *Archives of Physical Medical Rehabilitation, 69,* 415–418.

Kernberg, O. (1976). *Object relations theory and clinical psychoanalysis.* Northvale, NJ: Jason Aronson.

Klein, G. (1976). *Psychoanalytic theory: An exploration of essentials.* New York: International Universities Press.

Koocher, G., & O'Malley, J. (1981). *The Damocles syndrome: Psychological consequences of surviving childhood cancer.* New York: McGraw-Hill.

Kovacs, M., & Feinberg, T. (1982). Coping with juvenile onset diabetes mellitus. In A. Baum & J. Singer (Eds.), *Handbook of psychology and health* (Vol. 2, pp. 165–212). Hillside, NJ: Erlbaum.

Kutner, N.G. (1987). Social ties, social support, and perceived health status among chronically disabled people. *Social Science and Medicine, 25,* 29–34.

LaPlanche, J., & Pontalis, J.-B. (1973). *The language of psycho-analysis.* New York: Norton.

Leary, W.E. (1995, October 11). Many heart patients failing to seize a lifeline. *The New York Times.*

Levenson, P.M., Pfefferbaum, B.J., Copeland, D.R., & Silverberg, Y. (1982). Information preferences of cancer patients ages 11–20 years. *Journal of Adolescent Health Care, 3,* 9–13.

Lourde, A. (1980). *The cancer journals.* San Francisco: Spinsters/Aunt Lute.

Luborsky, L. (1962). Clinician's judgments of mental health. *Archives of General Psychiatry, 7,* 407–417.

Malan, D. (1976). *The frontier of brief psychotherapy: An example of the convergence of research and clinical practice.* New York: Plenum Press.

Mann, J. (1973). *Time-limited psychotherapy*. Cambridge, MA: Harvard University Press.

McCrae, R.R., & John, O.P. (1992). An introduction to the five-factor model and its applications. *Journal of Personality, 60*, 175–215.

McDaniel, S.H., Hepworth, J., & Doherty, W.J. (1992). *Medical family therapy*. New York: Basic Books.

McWilliams, N. (1994). *Psychoanalytic diagnosis: Understanding personality structure in the clinical process*. New York: Guilford Press.

Meeks, J.E. (1986). *The fragile alliance: An orientation to the psychiatric treatment of the adolescent* (3rd ed.). Malabar, FL: Robert E. Krieger.

Messer, S.B., & Warren, C.S. (1995). *Models of brief psychodynamic therapy: A comparative approach*. New York: Guilford Press.

Meyer, A.A., & Lewis, D.D. (1994). *Child with chronic illness* (Monograph No. 182). Kansas City, MO: American Academy of Family Physicians.

Morrow, G.R., Hoagland, A., & Carnrike, Jr., C.L.M. (1981). Social support and parental adjustment to pediatric cancer. *Journal of Consulting Clinical Psychology, 49*, 763–765.

Murphy, L.B. (1974). Coping, vulnerability, and resilience in childhood. In G.V. Coelho, D.A. Hamburg, & J.E. Adams (Eds.), *Coping and adaptation*. New York: Basic Books.

Newacheck, P.W., & Taylor, W.R. (1992). Childhood chronic illness: Prevalence, severity, and impact. *American Journal of Public Health, 82*, 364–371.

Pine, F. (1991). *Drive, ego, object and self*. New York: Basic Books.

Power, P.W., Dell Orto, A.E., & Gibbons, M.B. (Eds.). (1988). *Family interventions throughout chronic illness and disability*. New York: Springer.

Pynoos, R.S. (1990). Post-traumatic stress disorder in children and adolescents. In B. Garfinkel, G. Carlson, & E. Weller (Eds.), *Psychiatric disorders in children and adolescents* (pp. 48–63). Philadelphia: W.B. Saunders.

Rait, D., & Lederberg, M. (1990). The family of the cancer patient. In J.C. Holland & J.H. Rowland (Eds.), *Handbook of psychooncology: Psychological care of the patient with cancer*. New York: Oxford University Press.

Redd, W.H. (1990). Behavioral interventions to reduce child distress. In J.C. Holland & J.H. Rowland (Eds.), *Handbook of psychooncology: Psychological care of the patient with cancer* (pp. 573–581). New York: Oxford University Press.

Rolland, J.S. (1987). Chronic illness and the life cycle: A conceptual framework. *Family Process, 26*, 203–221.

Rowland, J.H. (1989). Interpersonal resources: Social support. In J.C. Holland & J.H. Rowland (Eds.), *Handbook of psychooncology: Psychological care of the patient with cancer*. New York: Oxford University Press.

Schulz, R., & Rau, M.T. (1985). Social support through the life course. In S. Cohen & S.L. Syme (Eds.), *Social support and health* (pp. 129–149). San Diego, CA: Academic Press.

Sigal, L.H., Adelizzi, R.A., Dato, V., Davidson, R., Frank, E.J., Genese, C., Murillo, J.L., Patella, S.J., Pellmar, M.B., Sensakovic, J., & Weisfeld, N.E.

(1993). *The New Jersey Lyme disease syllabus.* Lawrenceville, NJ: The Academy of Medicine of New Jersey.

Small, L. (1979). *The briefer psychotherapies* (rev. ed.). New York: Brunner/Mazel.

Stern, M.J., Pascale, L., & Ackerman, A. (1977). Life adjustment postmyocardial infarction: Determining predictive variables. *Archives of Internal Medicine, 137*, 1680–1685.

Stolorow, R.D., & Atwood, G.E. (1979). *Faces in a cloud: Subjectivity in personality theory.* Northvale, NJ: Jason Aronson.

Stone, M. (1993). *Abnormalities of personality: Within and beyond the realm of treatment.* New York: Norton.

Strupp, H., & Binder, J. (1984). *Psychotherapy in a new key: A guide to time-limited dynamic psychotherapy.* New York: Basic Books.

Stuber, M., Christakis, D., Housekamp, B., & Kazak, A. (1996). Posttrauma symptoms in childhood leukemia survivors and their parents. *Psychosomatics, 37*, 254–261.

Suinn, R. (1990). *Anxiety management training.* New York: Plenum Press.

Suinn, R. (1996, January 9). Anger: A disorder of the future, here today: Part 2. Treatment. *The Alaska Psychologist,* 11.

Sutkin, L.C. (1984). Introduction. In M.G. Eisenberg, L.C. Sutkin, & M.A. Jansen (Eds.), *Chronic illness and disability through the life span: Effects on self and family* (pp. 1–4). New York: Springer.

Taylor, S.E., & Aspinwall, L.G. (1990). Psychosocial aspects of chronic illness. In P.T. Costa, Jr., & G.R. VandenBos (Eds.), *Psychological aspects of serious illness: Chronic conditions, fatal diseases, and clinical care* (pp. 7–44). Washington, DC: American Psychological Association.

Weisman, A.D., & Worden, J.W. (1975). Psychological analysis of cancer deaths. *Omega: Journal of Death and Dying, 6*, 61–75.

Wenger, N.K., Froelicher, E.S., Smith, L.K., et al. (1995). *Cardiac rehabilitation* (Clinical Practice Guideline No. 17, AHCPR Publication No. 96-0672). Rockville, MD: U.S. Department of Health and Human Services.

Wertlieb, D.L., Jacobson, A., & Hauser, S. (1990). The child with diabetes: A developmental stress and coping perspective. In P.T. Costa, Jr., & G.R. VandenBos (Eds.), *Psychological aspects of serious illness: Chronic conditions, fatal diseases, and clinical care* (pp. 65–95). Washington, DC: American Psychological Association.

Whitt, J.K. (1984). Children's adaptation to chronic illness and handicapping conditions. In M.G. Eisenberg, L.C. Sutkin, & M.A. Jansen (Eds.), *Chronic illness and disability through the life span: Effects on self and family* (pp. 69–91). New York: Springer.

Zetzel, E. (1968). The so-called good hysteric. *International Journal of Psycho-Analysis, 49*, 256–260.

Worksheets

The Medical Template

OUTCOME: What is the outcome of the disease?

PROCESS: What is the disease process?

ETIOLOGY: What is the etiology of the disease?

NEEDS: What are the expected management needs?

The Threat Template

LIFE-THREATENING: The disease poses a significant threat to life.

PROGRESSIVE: The disease is understood but is progressively disabling.

UNPREDICTABLE: The disease is poorly understood and unpredictable in its course.

MANAGEABLE: The disease is understood and manageable.

The Response Template

INITIAL RESPONSE: Something is wrong.

AWARENESS OF CHRONICITY: Something continues to be wrong.

DISORGANIZATION: Whatever is wrong is disturbing my life in significant ways.

INTENSIFIED WISH FOR A CURE: Whatever is wrong must be changed.

ACKNOWLEDGMENT OF HELPLESSNESS: I cannot change what is wrong.

ADAPTATION TO ILLNESS: How can I live with what is wrong and is changing my life?

The Psychological Template

REALITY: How does the person manage reality?

ANXIETY: How does the person manage anxiety?

RELATIONSHIPS: How does the person manage relationships?

COGNITION: How does the person manage cognition?

MASTERY–COMPETENCE: What is the person's mastery–competence level?

Author Index

Subject Index

About the Authors

Carol D. Goodheart, EdD, is a psychologist and psychoanalyst who practices in New Jersey. She is the president and chief executive officer of PsychHealth, P.A., a multispecialty independent group practice corporation, which specializes in health psychology and offers treatment services, program design, consultation, and outcome research. She is also a clinical supervisor for the Graduate School of Applied and Professional Psychology at Rutgers University and a faculty member of the Institute for Psychoanalysis and Psychotherapy of New Jersey. Dr. Goodheart is the co-chair of the American Psychological Association's (APA) Congressional Initiative on Serious Illness; senior advisor for the APA Genetic Susceptibility Project; an APA Fellow; and a member of the New Jersey Breast and Cervical Cancer Control Coalition. She was given the New Jersey Psychological Association's Psychologist of the Year Award in 1991 for her distinguished contributions to the science and profession of psychology. Dr. Goodheart teaches, writes, lectures, and does psychotherapy with people who have serious medical problems, such as cancer, heart disease, and diabetes.

Martha H. Lansing, MD, practices both family medicine and psychotherapy. She is a Diplomate in the American Board of Family Practice, and she is certified in psychoanalytic psychotherapy by The Institute for Psychoanalysis and Psychotherapy of New Jersey. Dr. Lansing is a clinical assistant professor in the Department of Family Medicine at Robert Wood Johnson Medical School in The University of Medicine and Dentistry of New Jersey. She is the associate director of the Family Practice Residency Program at Helene Fuld Medical Center, and she directs the residency program's teaching practice, the Family Health Center.